FITNESS OVER 40

Robert Poyton

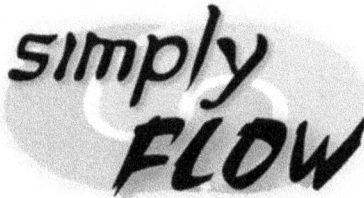

simply
FLOW

Published by Cutting Edge

ISBN: 9781645162636

*"We don't stop playing because we grow old;
we grow old because we stop playing."*
- George Bernard Shaw

CONTENTS

CHAPTER ONE

FUNDAMENTALS

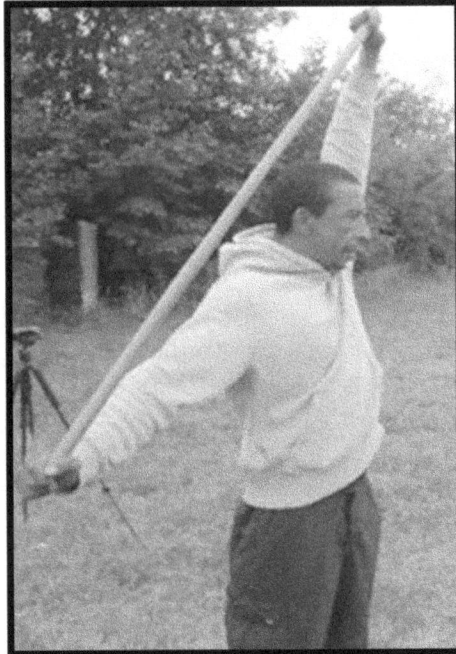

INTRODUCTION

I turned 50 a few years back, five years in fact, at the time of writing. I found that a lot of friends around the same age began asking me about the best way to keep fit and active as they got older. Now, I've been engaged in martial arts and health training since I was a young boy, so I have my own long-established training methods, developed over the years. But for people without a fitness background, what is the best approach to take?

I started looking around at various on-line training courses to see what was out there. To my surprise, virtually every one I checked out was concerned with just one particular aspect of fitness - how you look. The emphasis was solely on body sculpting, developing a six-pack, posting selfies on Facebook of the "new you."

All well and good, if that is what you are after. But this approach, to my mind, is rather shallow and it also misses out on two fundamental aspects of fitness, both of which become increasingly important as we age: mobility and tension.

Mobility, in brief, is our ability to move and operate as a fully functional human being. Barring injury, disease or disability, there is no real reason why we should not be as mobile at 70 as we were at 7. That may seem like a bold statement but I stand by it. The reason that many people are not so mobile is down to the second aspect, tension.

Tension has many causes, psychological and physical. Stress, worry and concern, be it about money, relationships or just from reading the news, have a much bigger impact on our health and fitness than we think. Prolonged exposure to even low levels of stress has a detrimental effect on our immune system, creates muscular tension throughout the body, affects sleep patterns and can have a negative impact on our work and relationships.

Physical tension can result from poor posture, lifestyle habits, injury, lack of activity, or doing the wrong type of activity. Some fitness methods actively introduce more tension into the body, which can result in problems. Remember the "feel the burn" fitness fads from a while back? Or some of the current big name fitness methods which encourage people to constantly go fast and hard? Visually impressive from a marketing point of view, but potentially physically damaging.

THE SIMPLY FLOW PROGRAM

With that in mind, I designed a program based on specific criteria:

- to be suitable for people with little or no fitness experience;
- to be efficient and effective;
- to be simple and natural;
- must be safe to practice;
- to help rediscover youthful freedom of movement and sense of play;
- to improve the overall health and well-being of the practitioner.

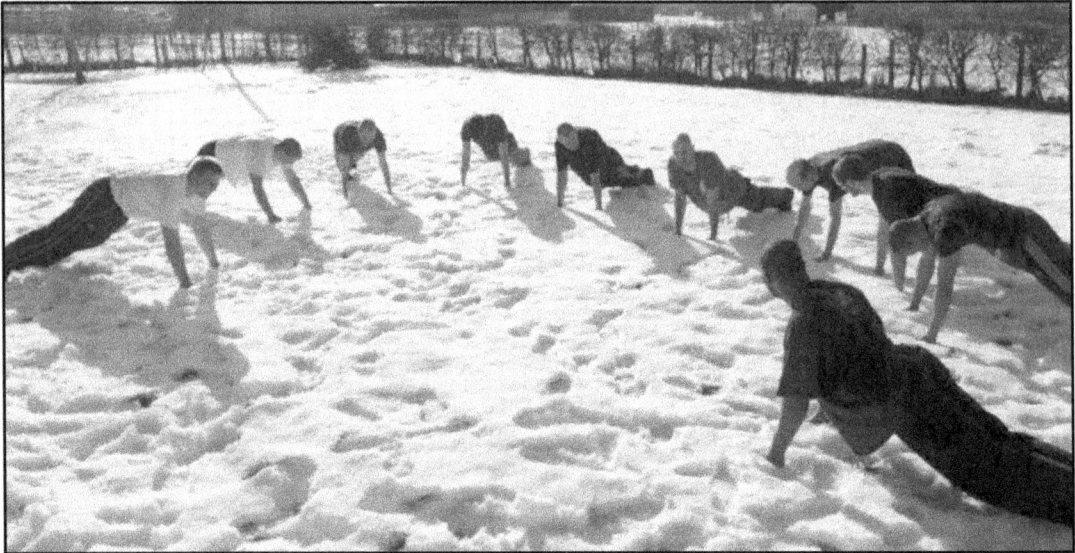

The basis for the program was my extensive training in Chinese and Russian martial arts, along with associated health practices. People are sometimes surprised that martial arts incorporate health and fitness training but consider that an unhealthy warrior is a warrior unable to fight! Most martial traditions have parallel systems of massage, medicine, and even stress control. War is one of the most stressful experiences a human being can go through, dealing with its after-effects was part of many warrior traditions, something that to a large extent has been sadly lost in modern times.

Having put the *Simply Flow Online Training Program* together, I tested it with a group of willing volunteers, before releasing it to the general public. Subscribers to the program received a weekly e-mail linking to five short video lessons per week, each showing a different exercise, or routine. Several people also asked if the program was available in book form and the answer is now, yes! I am also compiling those video lessons into specific downloadable modules for those looking for "bite size" training.

HOW TO USE THIS BOOK

I advise you work through this book chapter by chapter and get a good feel for the exercises. There is no need to rush any of the movements and this is not a "numbers based" system. By that I mean that the emphasis is on quality rather than quality. You will get more benefit from doing five real push ups than thirty of the "apple-bobbing" variety.

If there are any exercises that you feel uncomfortable doing, or that do not suit your current condition, then feel free to give them a miss. If at any time you feel pain or severe discomfort while doing an exercise, then please cease it immediately.

If in doubt, always check with your Doctor before trying any new exercise plan. If you have an existing medical condition or injury, then work within its restrictions, do not attempt to "blast through" it. Many of the exercises here can adapted to suit most conditions with a little thought. Of course, they can also be adapted to be made more challenging, once we have some experience!

But before we get there, it is very important that we have good basics. Any building is only as strong as the foundations, in our case what we call the *Four Pillars*. More about those in a minute. In short, work through the exercises at a steady pace, follow the instructions carefully and listen to your body. This program is designed to be long term, not a quick fix exercise plan. It is designed to incorporate natural human movement, movements that will carry over into your everyday life and activities. Use it wisely and I'm sure you will enjoy a healthy and active life for many years to come!

THE FOUR PILLARS

All of our work in the Russian martial art of *Systema* (a major source for this program) is based around the concept of Four Pillars. I think of these as the four legs of a chair, each must be present and of the right length, otherwise we wobble! The Pillars are: breathing, posture, relaxation/tension and movement. The four are, of course, closely inter-related, but to keep things clear, let's first examine each in turn.

BREATHING

The most fundamental Pillar, for without breath there is no life! We can go without food and water days or weeks, but most people struggle to hold their breath for even a couple of minutes. Breathing is a largely unconscious activity which goes on 24/7 and that is where the problems begin. We lose touch with our breathing and, consequently, it becomes less effective and efficient as we age. Again, medical conditions aside, there is no need for this to happen. Re-establishing conscious contact with our breathing is the first step to improved health and fitness.

The breath also acts as a very strong two-

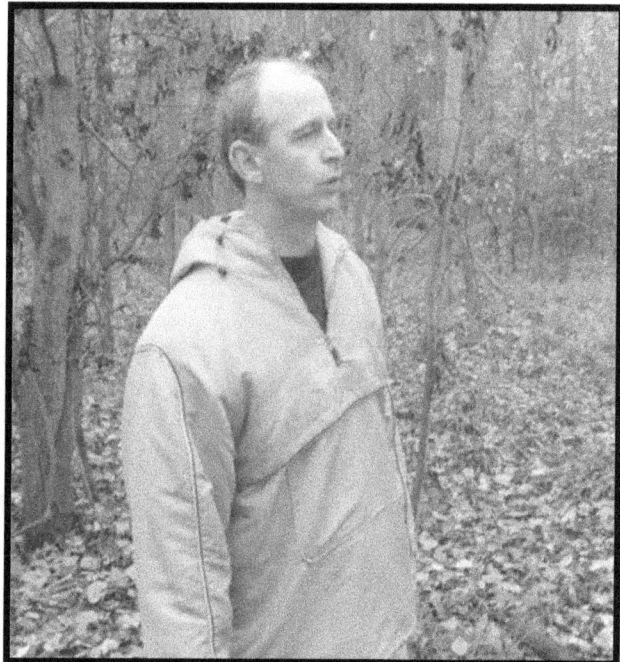

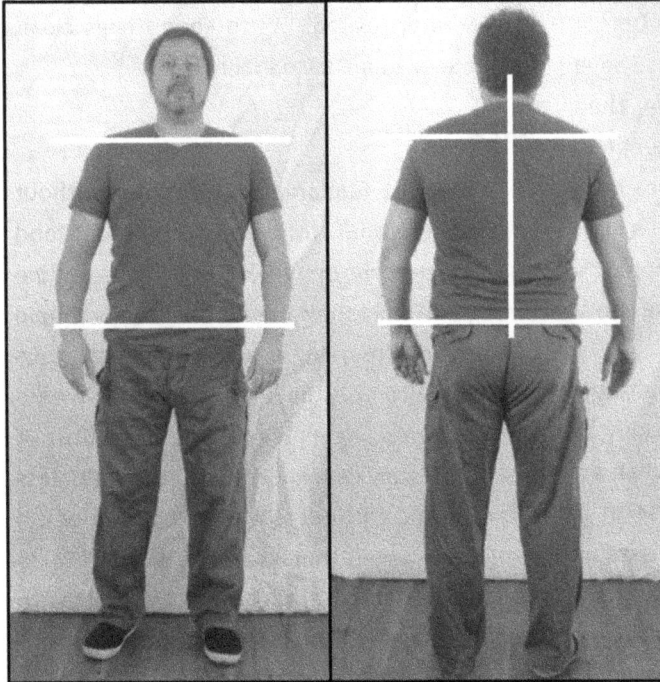

BALANCED POSTURE
Shoulder and hips level
Spine straight

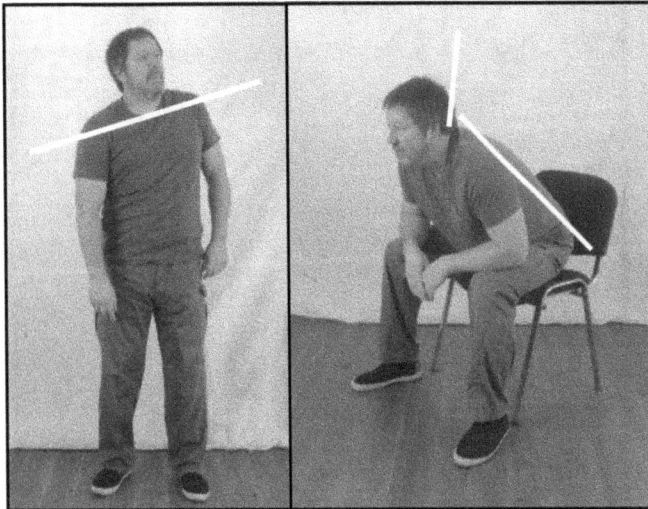

POOR POSTURE
Shoulders tense
Neck bent, body leaning

way bridge between our internal/emotional state and our external / physical state. When used correctly, the breath connects the two and allows one to influence the other. This makes breath work our primary method of stress management and fear control. Breathing can also be used to power movement.

POSTURE

Watch how a baby or toddler sits, watch how they squat or move up and down from the floor. You will notice they have a perfectly straight back and very open hips. As we grow older, posture often deteriorates. This can be due to injury and illness but is more often down to lifestyle, tension and general bad habits.

Improved posture means we move better, breathe better and place less stress on our joints. It can also help with back issues, which currently account for the loss of millions of working days in the UK.

Good posture simply means keeping the body in balance. It is not about "standing to attention" in a tense, military fashion, but simply maintaining a relaxed, neutral position - shoulders and hips level, spine straight. Check yourself in a mirror, check to see if your shoulders tilt. When you sit, try and keep the back upright and don't let the head tilt, as this can cause tension in the neck.

It is very good to get into the habit of monitoring your posture regularly throughout the day. If you are sitting at a desk for a long period of time, every now and then check that you are not hunching, leaning, or tilting the neck, for example.

RELAXATION

Relax is a very loaded word in the context of fitness. It usually conjures up images of sitting on the couch with a beer, not something that most fitness coaches condone! *Simply Flow* use the term relax more as a measure of how much tension there is in the body. Basically, we are always looking to operate with the minimal amount of tension necessary to complete the task.

Why? Because unwanted tension creates restriction and damage! Think of tension as salt. We need salt to survive, so we add a pinch here and there to our food. But too much salt creates problems, raises blood pressure and so on. Similarly, who would pour half a pot of salt onto their ice cream? We use it as and when necessary (although, of course, modern processed foods often contain much more salt and sugar than we are aware of.)

The same principle applies with tension. If the body is completely relaxed, it cannot move and we are laying on the floor. Even to stand takes a measure of tension. Yet how many people stand with buttocks clenched, hips tight, with a slight lean, shoulder raised, forehead creased in worry? And all you are doing is standing!

This kind of tension constricts breathing and blood flow and inhibits movement. When fast movement is carried out under tension, we run the risk of injury (as in the more

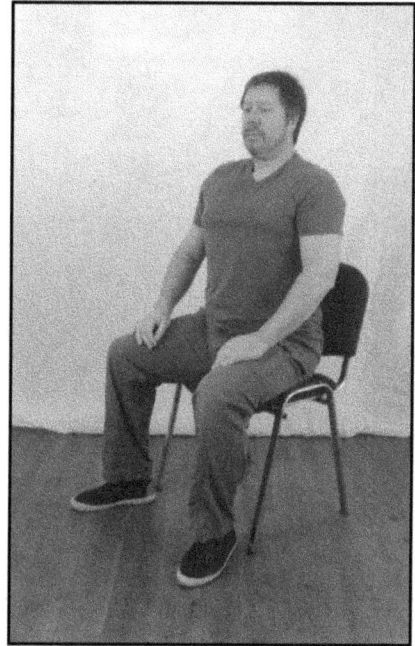

SITTING POSTURE
Spine straight,
shoulders relaxed

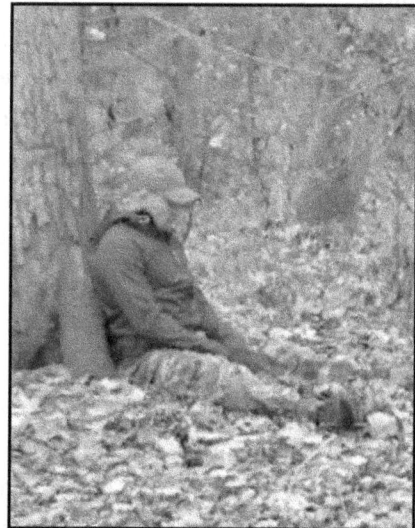

RELAXED SITTING
Outdoors environment

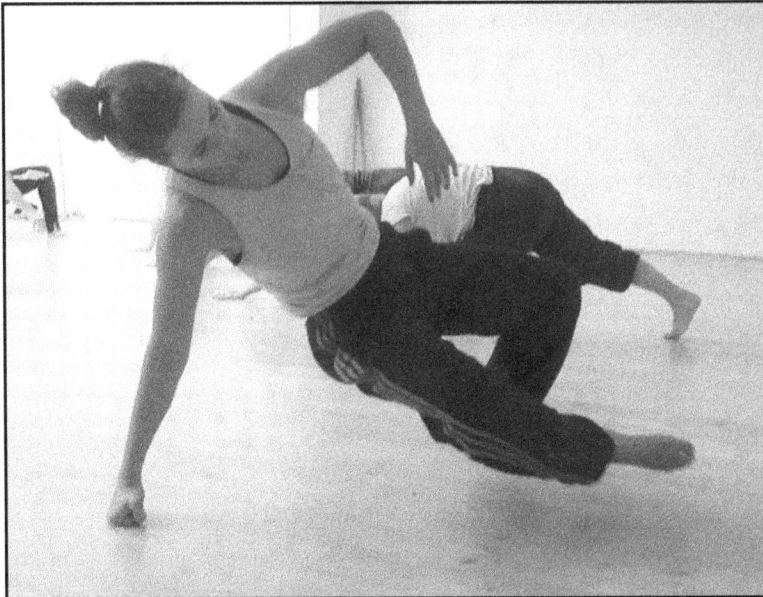

movement. As children we run, fall, climb, swim, jump and roll. There are very few inhibitions on our movement. As we grow older, those inhibitions grow. It may be that we drive to work, spend all day sitting at a desk, drive home again and sit on the couch all night. It may be that tension "freezes" our shoulders and they become more and more hunched.

dangerous forms of exercise).

Tension is closely related to posture and fixing one will usually fix the other. So again, get into the habit of monitoring tension levels throughout the day. That also includes your emotional tension - negative thoughts and stress contribute greatly to physical tension!

Learning to release tension and relax into our movement gives us efficiency and and flow. Watch how cats move in everyday activity, smooth and fluid. That brings us to our last Pillar.

MOVEMENT

Bio-mechanically, we are little different from the animals we share the world with, particularly mammals and apes. We take in information through our senses and interact with our environment through movement. Even speech is a function of breathing and

In short, use it or lose it! As I said before, medical reasons aside, there is no reason to have lesser mobility as we grow older. There are numerous studies that show how maintaining mobility reduces the effects of ageing. That includes good range of motion, flexibility, smoothness of movement, and so on.

Mobility is the ability to move ourselves in an efficient and effective way; a way that minimises impact and wear on the body but allows us to complete our task successfully, whatever it may be. Under the Simply Flow approach, there is no distinction in what you use your movement for, be it exercise, sports, dancing, swimming or just everyday activities, it is all the same process. Our exercise should be natural and free, so that our training truly prepares us for life!

INTEGRATION

When you practice each of the exercises, bear the Four Pillars in mind. Some exercises may focus specifically on one or two Pillars, in order to help understand them better but you should always be aware that they are holistic and inter-dependent. You can't breathe well with poor posture or if your posture is twisted! Work each Pillar step by step. Keep within your comfort zones to begin with, then gradually extend them.

There is what we could call a Fifth Pillar, which is the combination of all the other four working smoothly and efficiently together. Sports people often call this "being in the zone", some call it mindfulness, others the "flow state." Martial artists experience it as being "in the moment" and acting instinctually and powerfully in a dangerous situation. If you practice correctly and with diligence, I don't doubt that you will enter this state at certain times, particularly if you are under some kind of pressure, or even just involved in joyful movement.

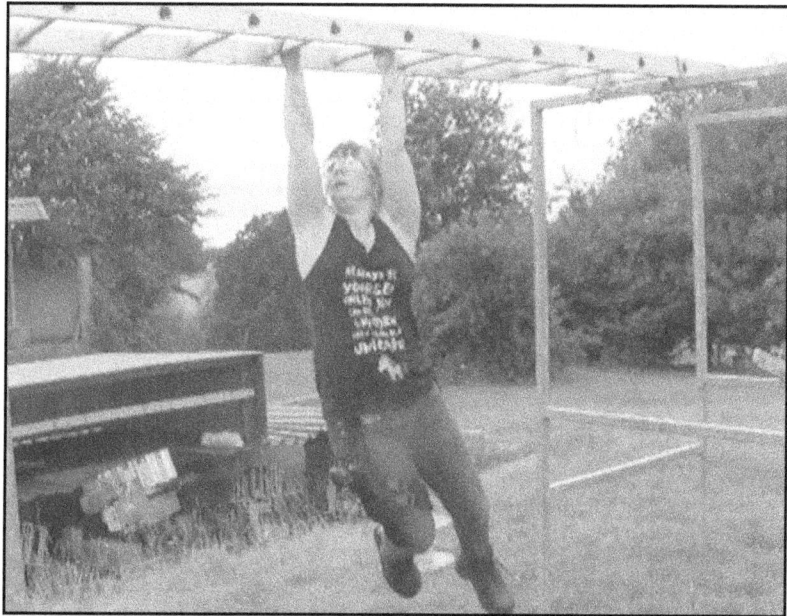

I use the word "joy" deliberately, though it is not something you often hear in the world of fitness. Everything is supposed to be "sweat, struggle and strain." Our view is that life has enough of those already, why spend your free time chasing them? Think back again to how children behave; they explore and interact, everything is new and exciting. They play, without any thought as to how they look and without any motive other than to enjoy themselves.

Apply the same feeling to your exercise. Learn to move and function with joy, it will have a profound effect on your life as a whole.

Let's begin!

CHAPTER TWO

BREATHING

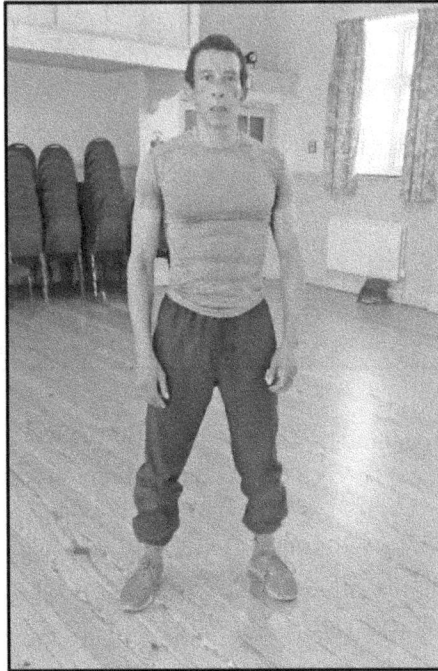

BREATHING

Unless otherwise directed, the standard breathing procedure is to inhale through the nose and exhale through the mouth. Breathing should be comfortable, not over filling the lungs or completely emptying them, unless otherwise directed. Learn to breathe smoothly and to the requirements of the situation. When you first start out, it is advisable to practice breathing in a safe and comfortable position. If you have any blood pressure or other health issues, always check with your healthcare professional prior to training.

DEPTH OF BREATHING

There are three basic depths of breathing. The first is shallow or burst breathing. Think of a dog panting, the breath comes in the nose and straight out of the mouth. This is most often used as a recovery breath, or in stressful situations. If your system is stressed you can use burst breathing to regain control and return to a state of equilibrium.

The second is our everyday chest breathing. The ribcage expands and contracts with each inhale and exhale. This may still be fairly shallow, or can be practiced more deeply. The main point to watch is that there is no unnecessary tension on the inhale, particularly in the shoulders.

The third is abdominal breathing, as used by singers and martial artists. This is where the diaphragm is fully used in order to draw and expel the breath. This can be "normal", where the diaphragm pushes out on the inhale, in on the exhale, or "reverse breathing" where the diaphragm pulls in and up on the inhale and expands out on the exhale.

We recommend you begin with chest breathing, with burst breathing for recovery. Deeper breathing will come with time as your body relaxes. Never force the breath and if at any time you feel dizzy, then come out of the exercise immediately and sit quietly to recover.

CIRCULAR BREATHING

The most basic breathing pattern is Circular Breathing. One half of the circle is an inhale, the other half an exhale. Each should be equal in length and depth. The main aim of CB is to put us back in touch with our breathing, to give us

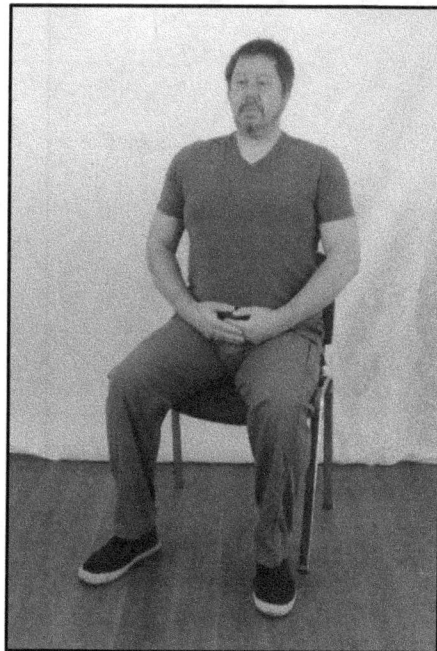

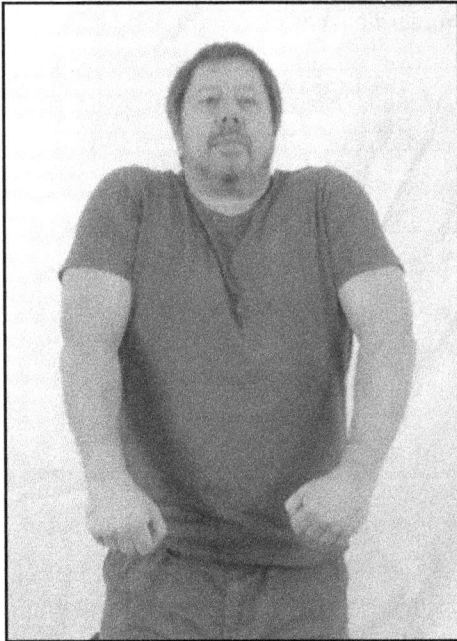

INHALE, TENSE

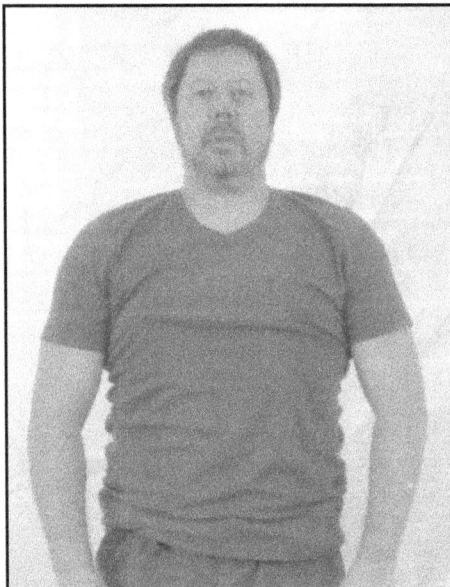

EXHALE, RELAX

conscious control over it.

Sit or lay down in a comfortable position. Relax the muscles, particularly around the shoulders. Now, in your own time, inhale to about 80% of your full capacity, then exhale the same. Don't worry about the length of breathing and be sure not to over-expand or tense the chest. Take around a dozen breaths in this position, keep it natural, keep it unforced.

You should find that even after a short exercise such as this you will feel a little more relaxed, both physically and emotionally. This, then, is an ideal exercise for those times during the day when we begin to feel stressed out. If you can, find yourself a quiet place and run through CB for a couple of minutes. This is also good preparation for situations such as going into an interview, having to speak in public, and so on. A minute or so of CB beforehand will help steady the nerves.

CIRCULAR BREATHING & SELECTIVE TENSION

Having worked one Pillar, let's add another. This time we will include a tense/relax cycle. The rule is we tense on the inhale, relax on the exhale. Selective Tension means that we only tense a particular muscle group, the rest of the body stays relaxed. In this case, we will work the shoulders.

Find a comfortable position, standing, sitting or prone. Inhale nose, exhale mouth for a while, slowing the breathing. Then, on the inhale, lift and tense the shoulders. Just the shoulders, remember! On the exhale, completely relax the shoulders. Repeat a few times.

Again, this is a great exercise to do as soon as you feel unwanted tension creeping into the shoulders - especially if you are sitting at a computer all day!

BURST BREATHING

The next thing to try is Burst Breathing, also sometimes called Recovery Breathing. This is where we inhale and exhale very quickly, almost like panting, so the breath is shallow and fast. We use BB in times of major stress, to help overcome fear and to quickly recover from being out of breath. In order to practice BB, we start by holding our breath.

Breath Holds tap into one of our strongest fears, the fear of not being able to breathe. Holding the breath also has many health benefits and, in some traditions the length of the hold is used as an indicator of your general health. You may be interested to hear that the current world record for holding the breath (without oxygen preparation) is over eleven minutes! That is quite an incredible feat of physical and mental discipline and obviously takes a huge amount of training - we will start with something a little easier!

Sit in a comfortable and quiet place. Inhale to about 80% capacity. Keep the body as relaxed as you can. You will soon feel tension build as fear kicks in and your body wants to exhale. Try and dissolve this tension, you can move the body a little or selectively tense and relax the muscles in question.

When you absolutely have to release the breath, do not take in a big gulp of air, but go into your BB. Short, shallow breaths to start, then gradually increase their length and depth until you are breathing normally again. You can repeat the same exercise with a hold on the exhale too.

Practice this exercise regularly and you will soon be able to hold your breath for two or three minutes with no problem. You will also find you get out of breath less often and when you do, you will be able to recover much quicker. Of course, BB is also another good method of settling nerves before, during or after a stressful event!

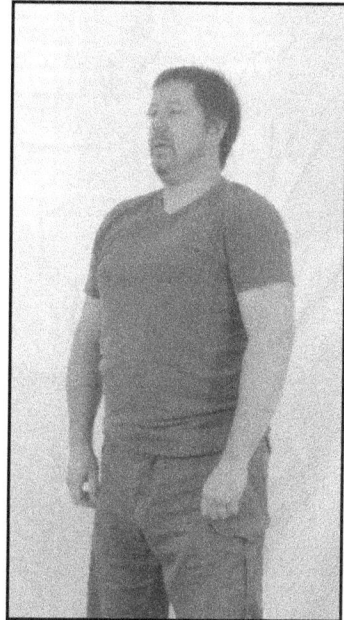

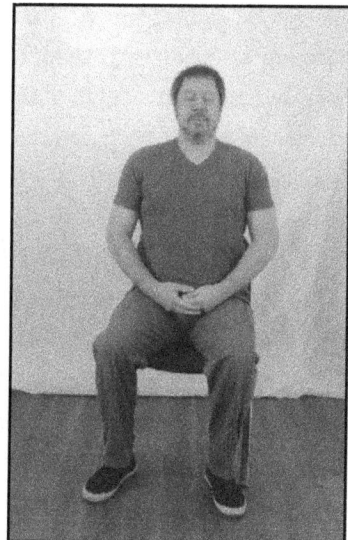

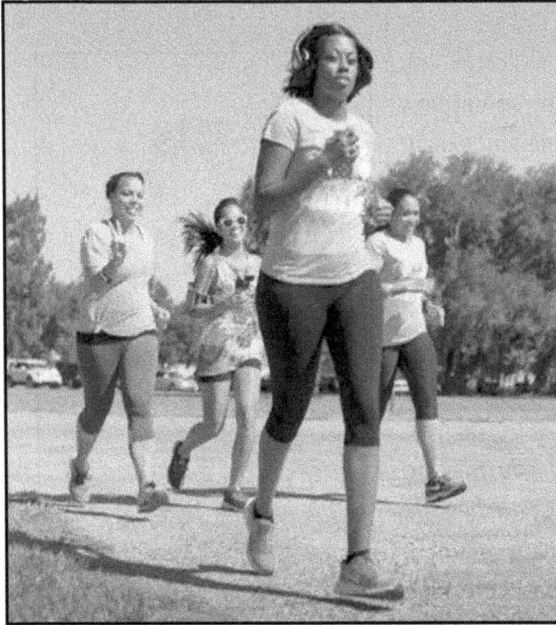

BREATH LADDERS

Once you are comfortable with CB, you can incorporate it into many activities, including walking and jogging. To do this, we use something called Breath Ladders. The idea is simple - we count the length of the breath, then gradually increase it, up to the top of the ladder, then back down again. Let's try a static version first.

Sit comfortably and begin CB. Keep the breaths short at first, say count to two on the inhale, two on the exhale. Do not try to take a quick, deep breath, keep the breathing shallow. After a few breaths, increase the count/length to four... then to six... then to eight. Each time the breath lengthens, it becomes a little deeper. Stay on eight for a while, then come back down the ladder,six, four, back to two, the breath

becoming shallow again. The amount of time you spend on each "rung" is up to you, depending on how much time you have. The top of the ladder is the length of breath you can still comfortably maintain, it may be six at first, or you may be able to go to ten. Again, over time your breath control and capacity will increase.

It's very easy to work the same exercise on the move. The count now becomes a number of steps. So a two count is two steps, increasing to four, six and so on. Once again, the inhale or exhale should spread smoothly across the steps. Work up the ladder, then back down again. If you practice this for a while, you will soon find a natural "groove" where your breathing and steps match perfectly. Stay in this and you will find a noticeable increase in your endurance, as your cardio system is now working very efficiently.

SQUARE BREATHING

Once you are confident with the Ladders, you can move on to Square Breathing. As the name implies, we now have four sides to the breath pattern - inhale, hold, exhale, hold. For now, we will keep each side an equal length. You can count in your head to being with.

Inhale as you count to four. Hold to the count of four. Exhale to four. Hold for four. That is one cycle. Of course, the number can be as low or high as you like. Practice SQ from a static position at first, then try it with the walking and jogging as above.

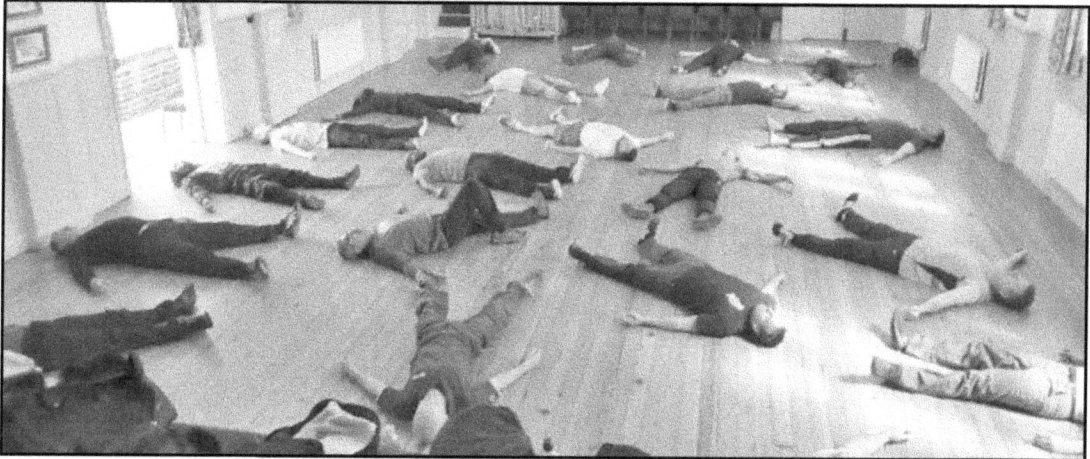

So that is Circle, Ladder and Square Breathing. Simple exercises it seems, they only take a few minutes to read but you should be aware that there is weeks and weeks of work contained within those straightforward drills! Do not neglect them and, of course, the advantage with breath work is that you can be practicing it almost anywhere.

Walking to the station? Ladders. Stressed because your train is late? Burst breath! On the train, Square Breathing for the duration of your journey. Even if it's only for five minutes a day, you will gain major benefits from these drills.

Also get used to monitoring your levels of stress and tension and deal with them straight away, or at least as soon as you can. If we can prevent stress getting a hold in the first place, it makes our work later on that much easier! Of course, these basic patterns can be added into most of the various exercises described later and that is something you can experiment with as you go along. As a starting point,

though, if no particular breathing pattern is described, then the default is to exhale on the exertion or the stretch. So for a push up, you inhale on the way down, then exhale on the way up. Once the pattern is comfortable, you can try to reverse the breathing sequence. The main thing is that you are breathing throughout!

In terms of timing, try and start the breathing just before the movement. This means that we learn to lead the movement with the breath, an important aspect of making our exercises mindful and not just robotic patterns. Remember to always keep your breathing smooth and even, even with the shallow breaths.

At the end of the book we will detail a complete, full body breathing exercise, as illustrated in the photo above. This is a great one to do at the end of a stressful day or if you just need a short break from the world!

CHAPTER THREE

MOBILITY

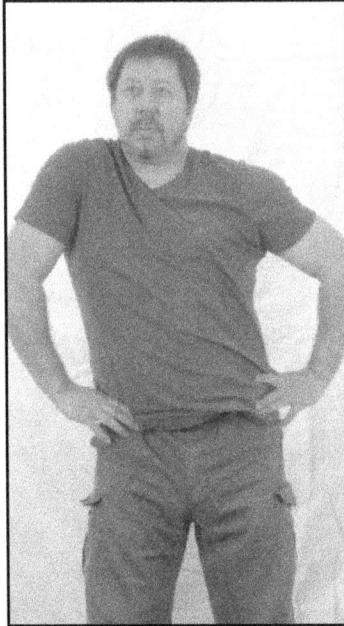

MOBILITY

Did you know that there are 360 joints in the human body? Now, a number of these are in places like the skull but even so, our bodies have marvellous articulation throughout and, in theory, we should all have an extensive range of motion (ROM). However, as we've already discussed, tension, fear and other factors often combine to limit our range of motion as we age.

The first step to restoring our freedom of movement is to establish our Comfortable Range of Motion (CRM). That is what these next series of exercises is designed to do. Once we have established the CRM we can work to extend it back out to its original scope.

We are going to start with the neck and go all the way down the body to the feet, working each of the major joints in turn. The first time you try this is purely to establish your CRM, so don't feel you have to make huge movements to start. Simply establish any problem areas and try to pinpoint where excess tension exists

At first, you don't even have to make circles, think about working in straight lines instead. Lift the shoulders up and down, for example, then back and forward, then you can make circles. At a more advanced stage, we can add in wave and spiral movement to develop our CRM even further.

Don't feel constrained to do only the movements presented here, begin to explore joint movement in as many directions as you can. Always stay relaxed when working the joints, don't place them under load and keep your movements smooth. There is no specific breathing pattern, unless noted.

The movements can be practiced standing or sitting (for the upper body part). Each movement should be repeated on each side, where appropriate - for reasons of space we have only shown one side. Repeat each movement a few times to get the feel of it.

BALANCE

Another benefit of CRM training for the legs is that we also improve our balance. To test your balance, stand in a relaxed position and raise one knee. It doesn't have to be high, as long as you have the foot off the ground. Are you steady or is there a wobble? If you are steady, you can try lifting your knee a little higher. If you are wobbling, there are three things to look at:

1. Posture - make sure the spine is straight, the shoulders and hips are level and the head is not tilted

2. Tension - typically, when people start to sway they tense in order to stop it. Tension only makes things worse! Relax the body, especially the shoulders and think about sinking down a little into the supporting leg.

3. Strength - the small stabiliser muscles are not up to the job. However even just standing one legged works the muscles on the supporting ankle and will strengthen them over time. Of course, you can use something for support if required.

HEAD AND SHOULDERS

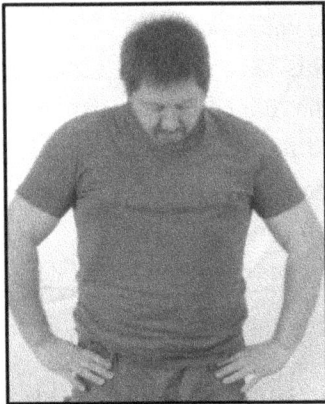

Drop the chin towards the chest. Pause for a second then lift the chin and tilt the head back.

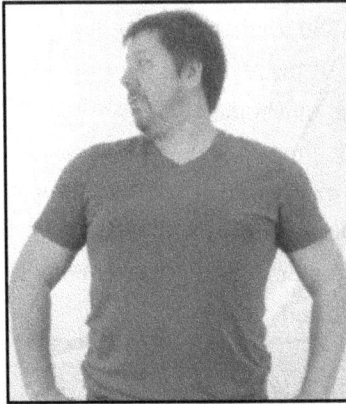

Turn the head slowly to look over the right shoulder, return to the middle, then look over the left shoulder.

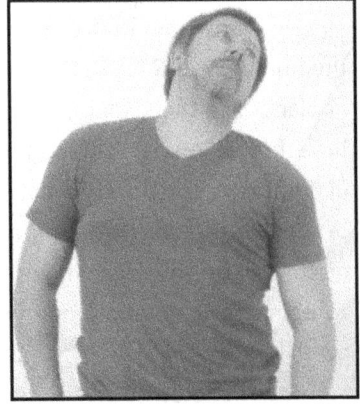

Drop the chin and rotate the head to the right. Stop and circle to the left. Keep the shoulders relaxed throughout.

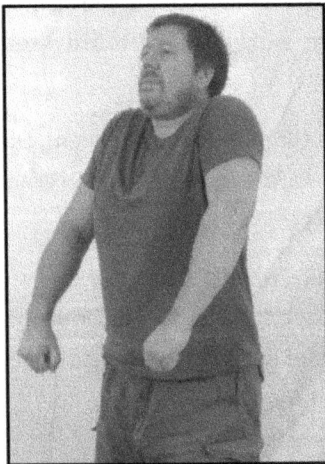

Inhale and lift the shoulders as high as you can. Exhale and let the shoulders drop.

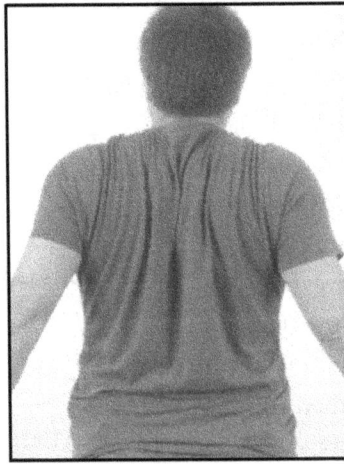

Inhale and squeeze the shoulder blades back together.

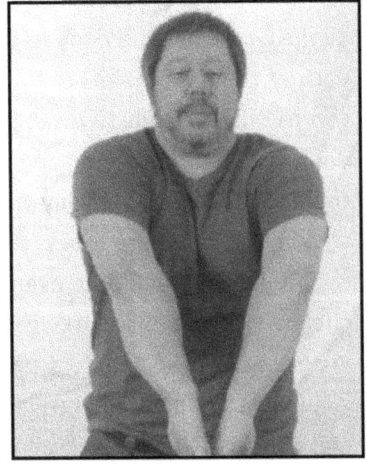

Exhale and open the back out - imagine you are trying to touch your shoulders together at the front.

ARMS AND HANDS

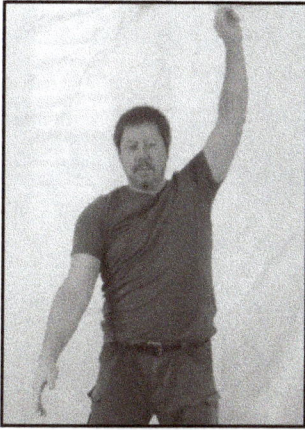

Begin with arms at the sides. Lift the hands and circle the arms backwards then forwards . Make a big circle, keep the arms straight but not locked.

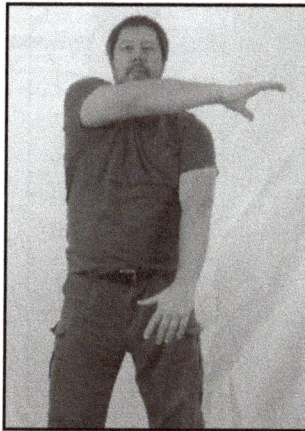

Start with hands at sides again. This time, circle the arms in front of the body . Make big circles, to the left and to the right.

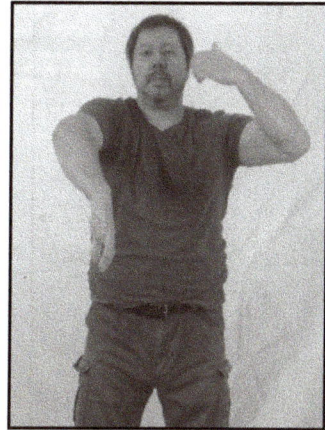

Raise the hands and circle the forearms from the elbow. Work in both directions.

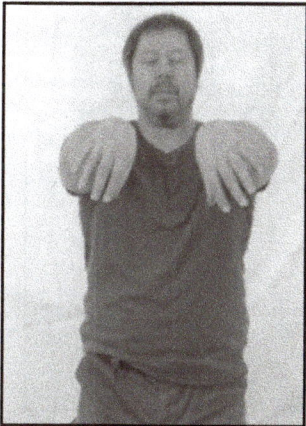

Hold your hands out in front. Relax the wrists and rotate them to the left and to the right.

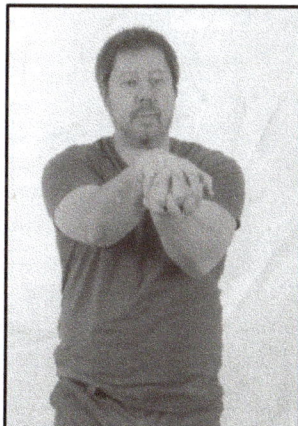

Clasp the fingers together and slowly roll the wrists around.

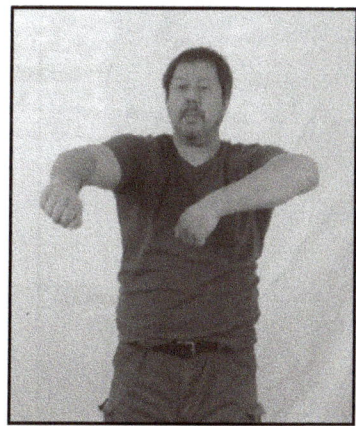

Circle each of the fingers and thumbs in turn.

TORSO AND HIPS

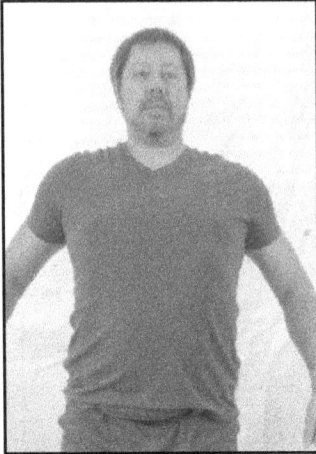

Inhale and expand the chest, exhale and let it sink.

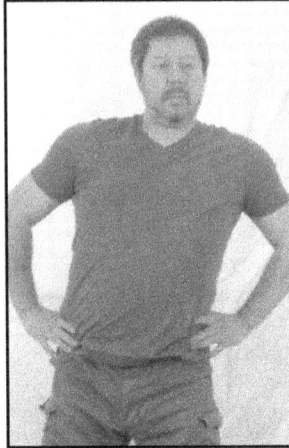

Keep the hips and shoulders as still as possible, move the rib cage to the right and left.

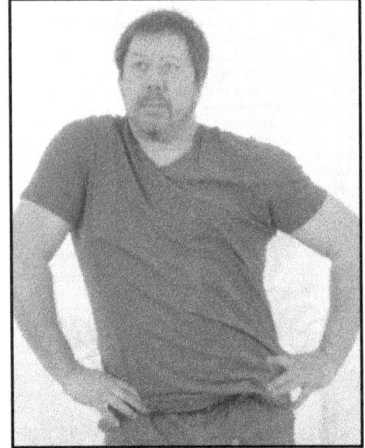

Circle the rib cage in both directions.

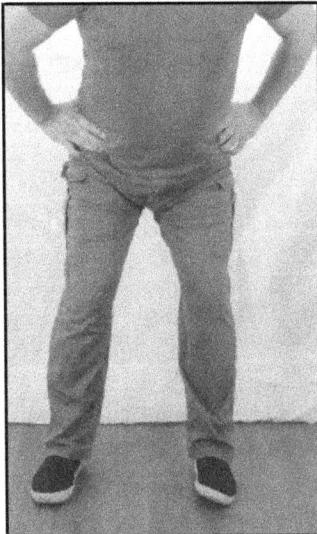

Swivel the hips backwards and forwards.
Keep the legs relaxed, do not lock the knees.

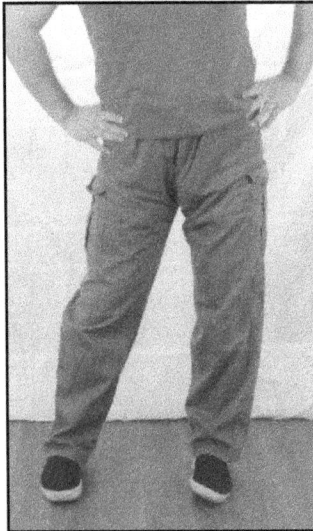

Repeat the same movement but this time swivel the hips left and right.

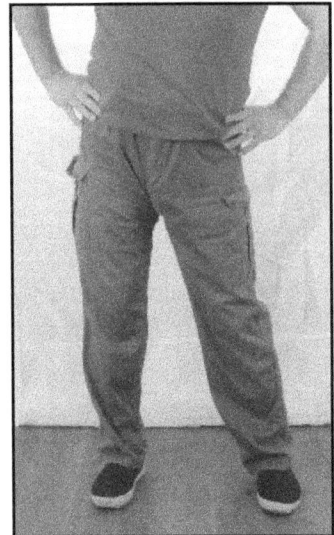

Now circle the hips in each direction. Once again, make sure to keep the legs relaxed.

LEGS

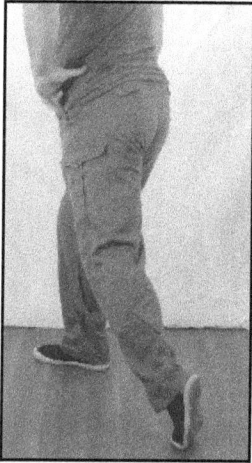

Place one foot forward, one back. Raise the heel on the rear foot and circle it, keeping the toes on the floor. Move the circle into the whole leg.

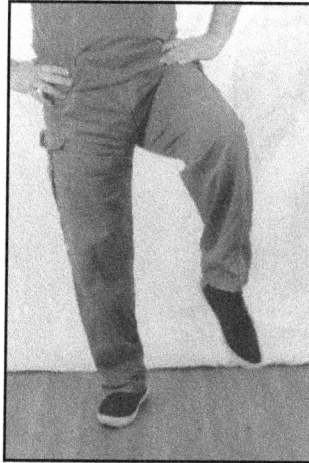

Lift one foot off the floor (use support if necessary.) Circle the ankle outward, then the knee, then the hip. Reverse the direction and repeat.

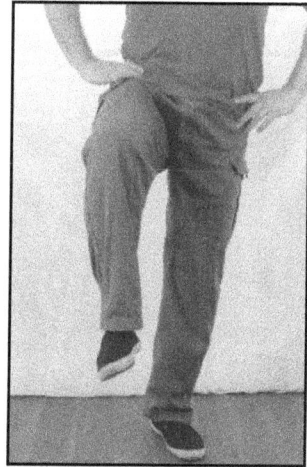

Lift a knee and circle the whole leg outwards. Keep the body straight. Place the foot down, then lift again and reverse direction.

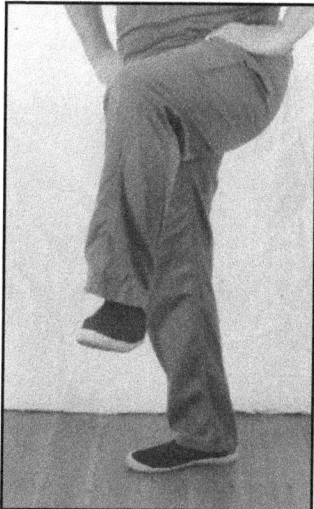

Raise the knee up in front.

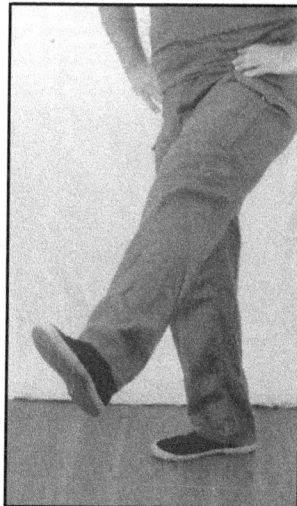

Push the foot forward and out.

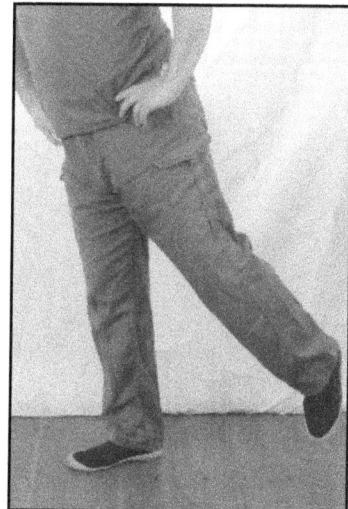

Swing the foot back. Try the movement in reverse too.

CHAPTER FOUR

CORE EXERCISES

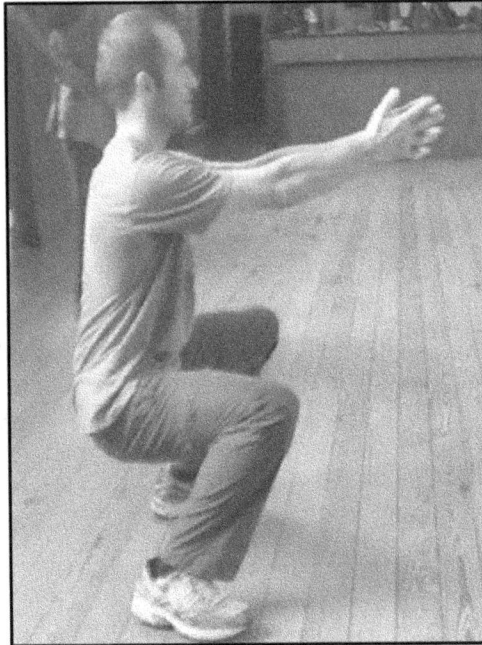

CORE EXERCISES

We call this next set of exercises our Core Exercises for two reasons. One, they are primarily about strengthening the core muscles of the body, in upper, middle and lower sections. Two, these three simple movements form the basis of all our bodyweight exercises. They are also the foundation for more advanced work, so it is important to practice them correctly.

On the face of it, the exercises are very simple. But simple should not be confused with easy! To practice any of these exercises, "perfectly" is a real challenge - and it is perfection we are after, not endless repetition.

Another point worth making is that when exercises like these are performed well, they not only strengthen the body but can also work to repair it. I had problems in both knees some years back, and spent three months doing squats with the assistance of a chair, to really fine tune my knee alignment. That was enough to rectify the issue. Of course, prevention is better than cure and these exercises will also help with that - a strong core is less susceptible to injury.

Our three exercises are the squat, push up and sit up. In each case we will show you preparatory exercises, helpful if you have not done these exercises before or require some assistance in doing them. Once you have the basic version of each exercise down, it is very easy to add in variations in order to make them more challenging. Later, I will explain how we can use a "formula" to achieve this. Not only does this provide more challenges for our body, it also stops the exercises becoming stale. Going through the same old routine over and over is boring, it's good to mix things up now and then!

As far as breathing goes for the CE, keep things simple to start. Inhale on one move, exhale on another. So, for a push-up, inhale down, exhale up (or vice-versa). The main thing is to keep breathing and not hold the breath, that will only bring tension into the body. The rhythm of the breathing also gives us a good indication of the speed that we should be working at. Not too slow, not too fast. We aim to keep the muscles under load for the full duration of the movement, so keep it smooth! Let's start with the squat.

THE SQUAT

In many parts of the world, people squat rather than sit. In fact, some in the West now describe sitting as the "new smoking!" As our lives become more sedentary, there is a danger that we lose mobility in the hips. If posture is fixed in a bad position, we misalign the spine. Extended sitting also means we lose strength in the legs. Some also claim that too much sitting around contributes to chronic health problems such as heart disease and diabetes.

Squats are a great exercise for keeping the hips open, for realigning the spine and for building leg strength. This is why the Chinese call the squats the "King of Exercises!" In traditional Chinese terms, strengthening the legs is also said to strengthen the heart and circulatory system.

I see many people practicing fast squats, again fixed on doing so many reps as quickly as possible. However, their posture is often all over the place (as shown in the picture above) and working this way will actually damage the body over time. So the first thing we need to do is establish our correct squat posture. We do this by practicing an "assisted squat", using the support of an object or other person to help get us into the correct position. Once your muscles get used to this position you will find doing a correct squat much easier.

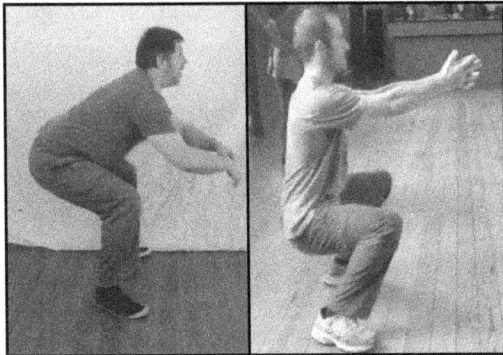

POOR AND GOOD SQUAT POSTURE

ASSISTED WALL SQUAT

Find a secure, flat surface, such as a wall or a closed door. Stand with your back to it. Bring the feet away from the wall a little and to a comfortable position, usually just over shoulder width apart. The toes must point in the same direction as the knees, they may be pointing straight forward, or be turned out a little, though not pointing inwards.

Inhale, then on an exhale, slowly bend the knees and lower yourself down. Just go to your comfortable range of motion at first. The trick is to maintain the alignment of the body, so the back should remain in full contact with the supporting surface, from shoulders to tailbone. If you tuck the tailbone in a little and tilt the

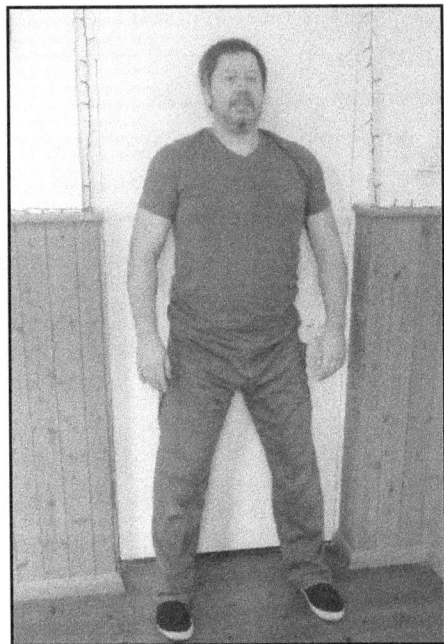

pelvis slightly, you will find it more comfortable. Hold for a second as you inhale, then exhale and straighten up again.

Repeat this a few times. As your strength builds and the hips open, you will be able to sink lower into the squat. You can also try going down into the squat and holding the position for a few minutes - this is a great one for the thigh muscles!

SQUATS

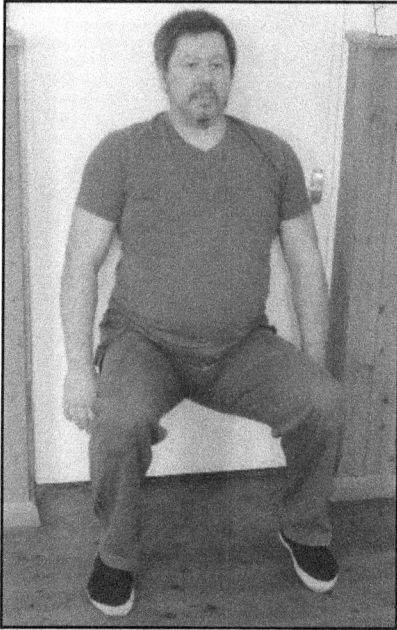

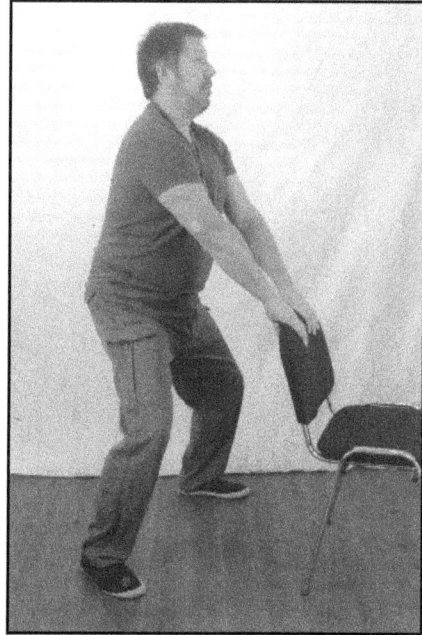

ASSISTED CHAIR SQUAT

You can work exactly the same exercise by using a chair or other stable object for support. This time, you grasp the object with your hands as your perform the squat. The accompanying photographs will give you some ideas about what you can use.

Always be sure that the object you use is stable and will support your weight. A heavy chair is good, or the edge of a table or counter. The same rules of body alignment apply, go slow and check yourself through each stage of the movement. If you find a "sticking point", then hold that position and try some burst breathing to relax the muscles.

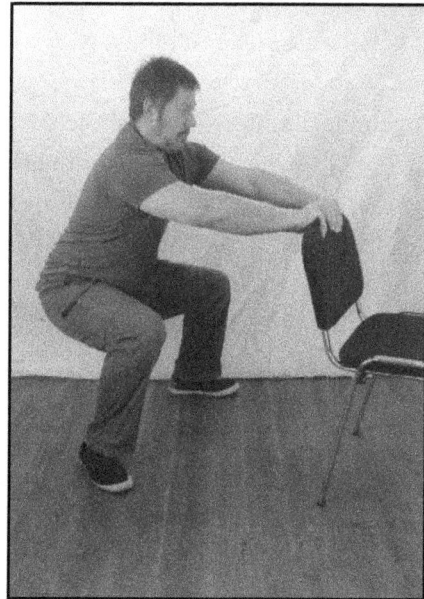

SQUATS

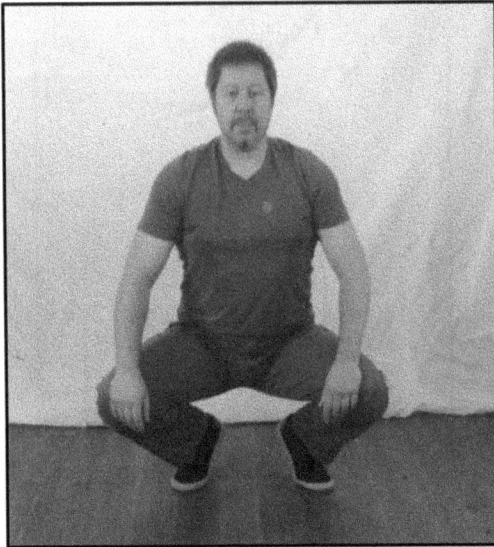

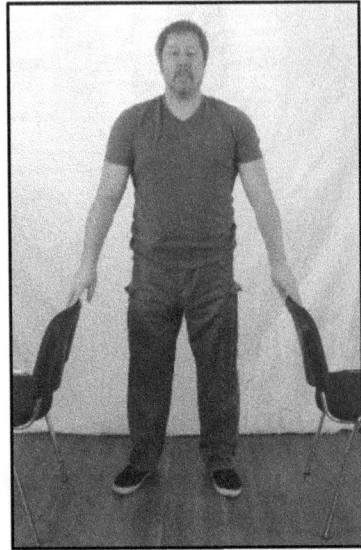

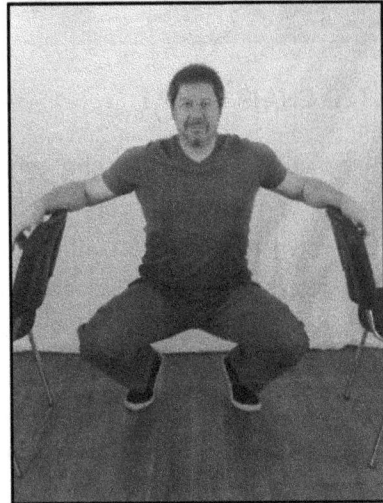

COSSACK SQUAT

If you have trouble squatting all the way down, or if you want to try an exercise that will help open the hips, take a look at the Cossack squat. The upper body is in exactly the same position as the conventional squat, but the toes point out for this one and the heels are raised. You should be able to work lower in this position. The Cossack Squat is also a foundation move for future Low Acrobatics and Ground Movement exercises.

You can begin with the assisted version, using either the wall or chair for support. Ensure, again, that knees and toes are in line. Inhale down, exhale up.

The Cossack Squat is also a great "resting" position. If you are involved in any activity and have to take a break for a minute, drop into the Cossack Squat. It will help keep your muscles loaded and is much better for you than sitting on the floor. In fact, I'd recommend you spend at least five minutes in the Cossack Squat everyday. Try it while you are watching TV or waiting for the kettle to boil!

SQUATS

THE FULL SQUAT

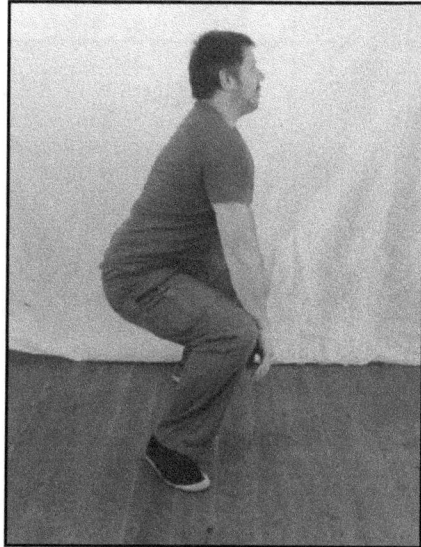

Once ready, try the full, unassisted squat. Get your stance comfortable, monitor your posture and slowly sink down. I prefer to keep the arms hanging down, but at first you may wish to extend them out in front for balance.

Remember it is better to go not so low and maintain good posture than to distort the posture to go lower. Check your alignments - knees and toes in line, spine straight, head not tilted, shoulders level, tailbone tucked slightly in. Inhale down, exhale up, with smooth movement

SINGLE LEG SQUAT

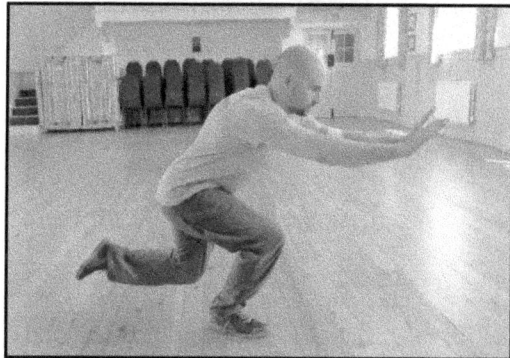

Once you feel comfortable with the standard unassisted squat, you can try working on one leg. The full version of this is known as the Pistol Squat , but to start, you can try this version, it is good preparation for the Pistol.

Start in the normal position, with feet a comfortable width. Inhale and start to squat down. As you do so push the hands forward and one leg back, as shown.

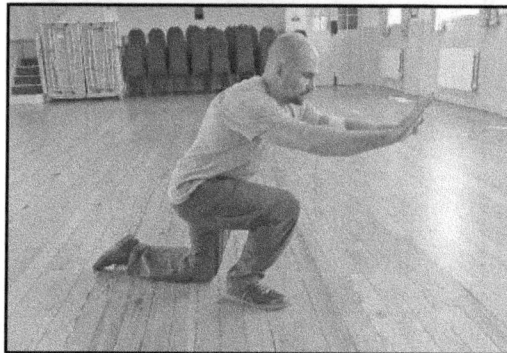

Take the rear knee all the way down to the floor. You may wish to work on a soft surface at first. Hold the position and take a couple of breaths. Then, as you exhale, push up from the forward leg, drag the back leg forward and return to standing position.

If you really want to train your balance too, then work this movement quite slow. Check your knee alignment throughout!

PUSH UPS

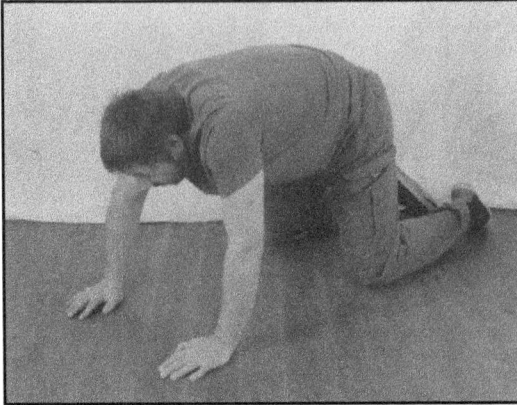

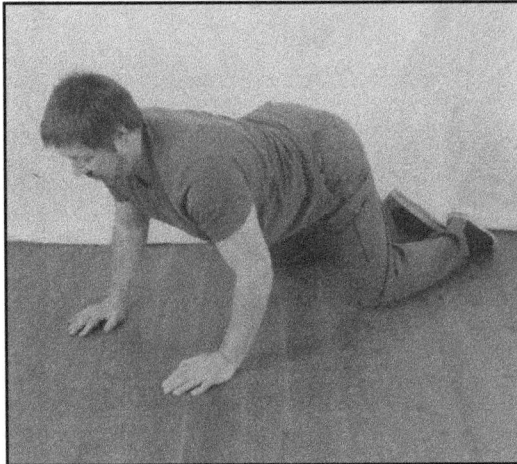

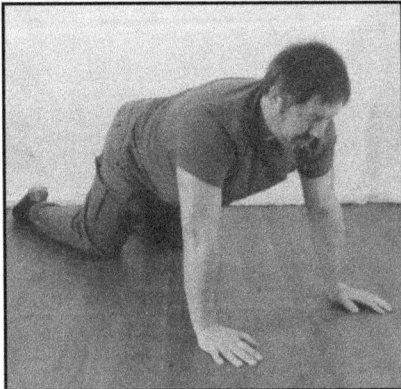

THE PUSH UP

The push up is a staple bodyweight exercise, one that almost everyone will have done some time in their life! All the same principles apply as with the squat, so let us first look at getting the correct posture, then some preparation exercises before doing the full push up.

Take up position on your hands and knees, hands under the shoulders. Rest your weight evenly on all four points of support. The main postural point to check is spinal alignment. In the first two pictures below see how the spine is first bowed upwards, and then how the spine is slumped, both producing a downward curve.

Both these positions are incorrect. What we are looking for is to maintain a level spine. Think of the back as a table - in the correct position you should be able to place things on it without them sliding off! In this way the spine supports the body fully and the core muscles will be correctly activated. This is also the start point for our first exercise.

PUSH UPS

THE POINTER DOG

Position yourself on all fours, hands under shoulders, knees under hips. Distribute your weight evenly in the hands and knees and keep the back level.

Without shifting your weight, raise your left hand and point it directly forward. Hold to a count of three, then return it to the floor. Now repeat the same movement with the right hand. The key point is not to shift weight in the hands and knees to compensate but to engage the core muscles to maintain stability.

Now repeat the same procedure with the feet. Lift the knee and point the toes straight back. Hold, then return, right and left.

Once you can hold each of these positions without wobbling, try all four movements as a complete sequence. Right hand, left hand, left foot, right foot , cycle the sequence round a few times. If you want to add in breathing, inhale on the floor, exhale on the point. Take your time and ensure that the back stays level to the floor.

Now try pointing hand and foot simultaneously. So right hand, left foot and vice versa. Extend and hold, return and switch sides.

When practicing this exercise, keep just the right amount of tension in the body. Too little and the body will sag, too much and you will find it hard to move the hands and feet. You'll soon get the correct feel.

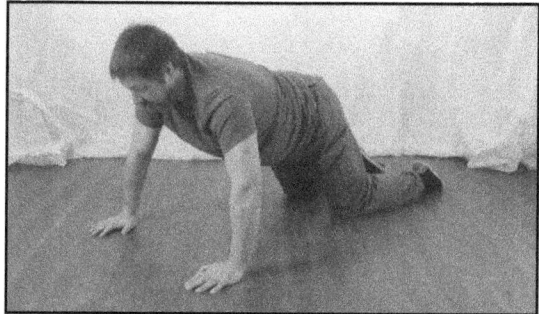

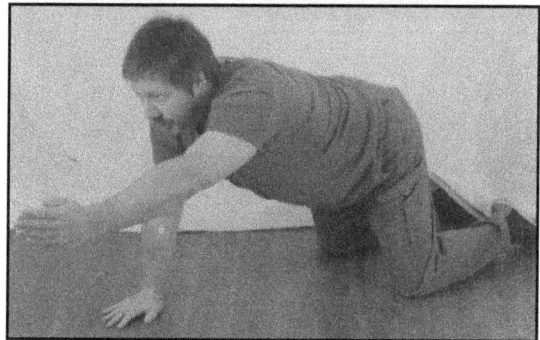

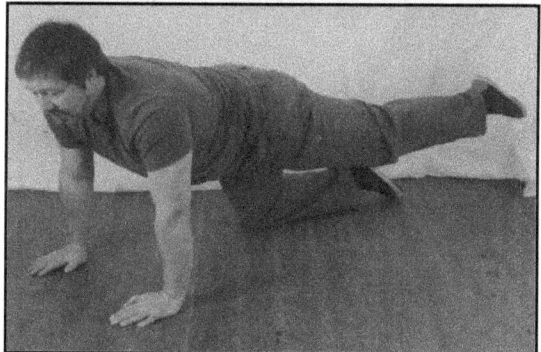

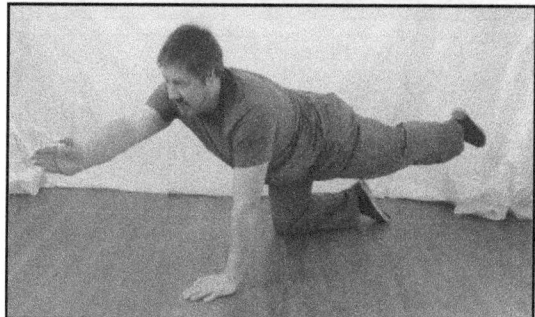

PUSH UPS

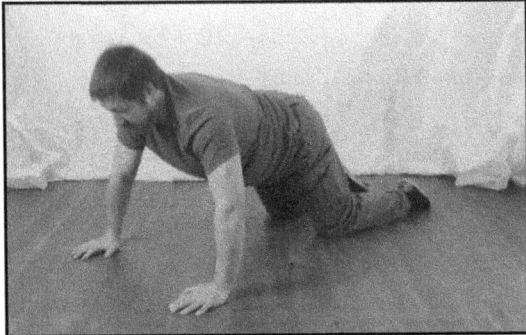

KNEE PUSH UPS

We can use the same start position for an assisted push up, with a slight adjustment. Move the hands forward a little in order to stretch the body out a little further.

From here, shift the weight forward into the hands. Now bend the elbows to bring the chest towards the floor. Go as low as you are comfortable with with at first. Inhale down, exhale up.

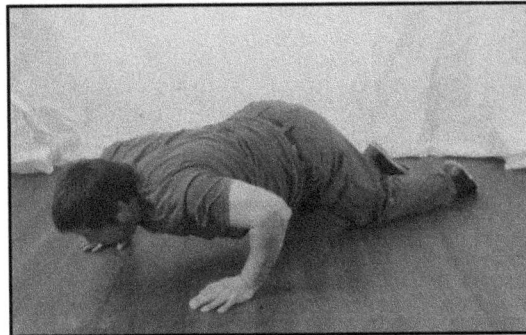

THE PLANK

The plank is, in effect, a static push up. It can be held at any point in the movement, we will start with holding at at the top. From the same start position as the previous exercise, take the feet back behind you. The hands are under the shoulders. You can rest on the palms or the fists, according to preference.

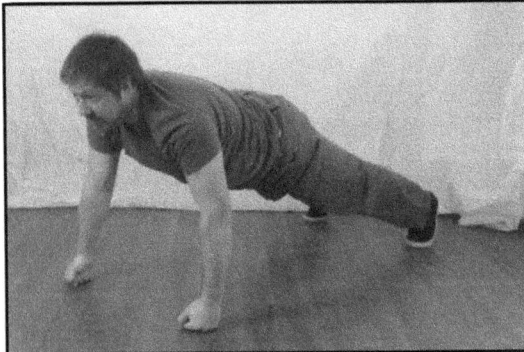

Some people like to maintain full body tension during the Plank. However, I want you to keep just enough tension in the body to prevent the back from sagging. Try and keep the shoulders and legs relaxed, remember to keep your breathing going, burst breathe if necessary. An alternative to using the hands is to rest the body on the elbows, as shown opposite.

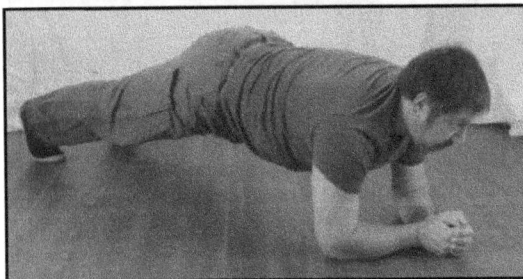

The amount of time you hold the Plank is up to you. First time round, see if you can make 30 seconds. You can gradually build up the time as you progress but remember, perfect form and relaxation is what we are after!

PUSH UPS

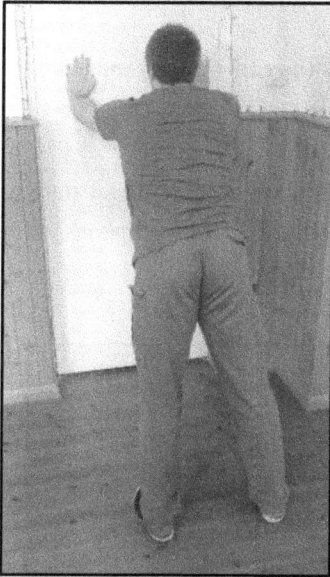 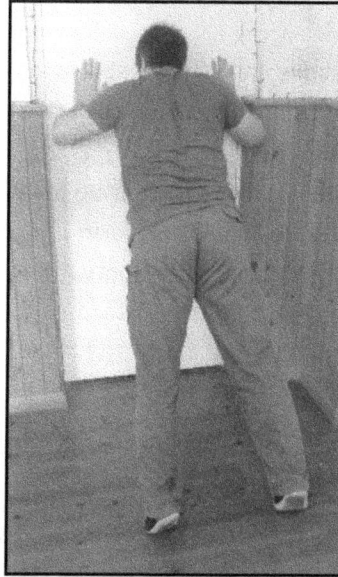

WALL PUSH UP

If you don't feel able to do a full push up yet, then you can also use the wall for an assisted push up. Place the palms on the wall and take the feet back a few steps. Now simply lean, lifting the heels and taking the weight of the body into the hands.

Inhale as you lean into the wall, exhale as you push yourself away. Be aware of spinal alignment again, no sagging!

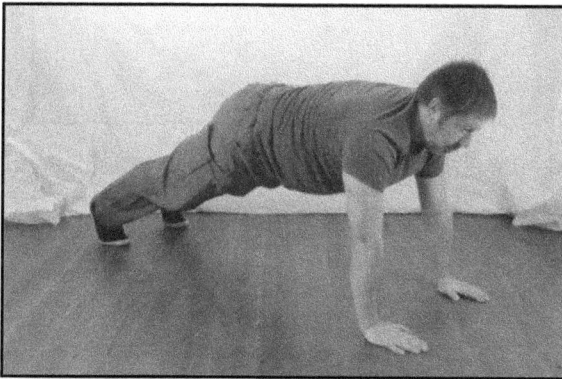

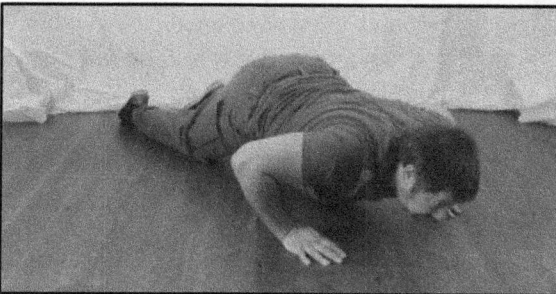

FULL PUSH UP

Start in the first plank position. Maintaining a level spine, inhale and lower yourself to the floor. Exhale and push back up. Try and keep shoulders, hips and legs relaxed.

In terms of speed, work at first to the length of your normal breath. Remember, start the breathing just before the movement. In terms of number of reps, set yourself a reasonable target to start and work to do each of those smoothly and with good posture. After that, work towards your upper limit, though not until failure. In other words, if you collapse at 15 push ups, then do 14. Then, as you improve, go to 16, etc.

SIT UPS

SIT UPS

Sit ups are another bodyweight staple and are a great way to work the central core and lower back. I would just add, if you have any back issues, then please exercise caution with some of these exercises, check with your doctor first!

One advantage of working on the floor is that we have much more support, so it is usually easier to maintain good posture. These exercises also form a good base for any future work we do on ground movement and mobility training. Let's start with something simple.

CRUNCHES

The simplest version of the sit up is a crunch. Lay on the floor, knees raised, hands behind the head. Inhale, then on the exhale lift the head up towards the knees. You don't have to lift very far. Inhale, return to the start position. You can experiment with lifting the feet and/or bringing the knees in as you lift the head too.

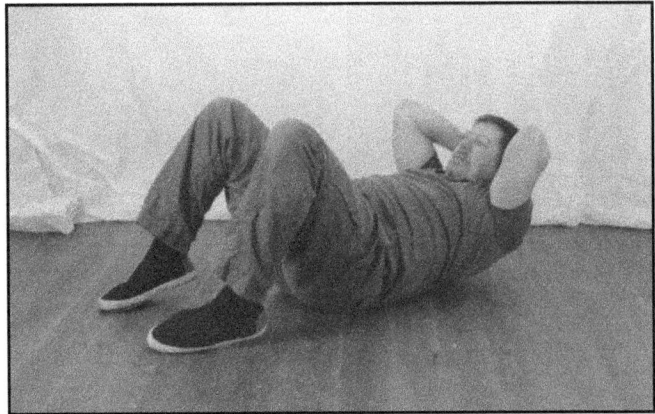

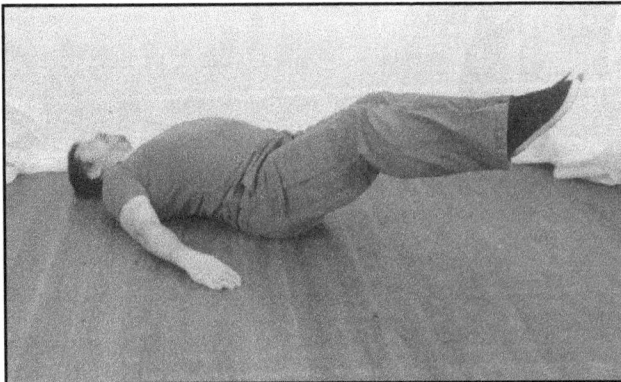

FOOT LIFT

Lay back, with arms at sides. Inhale, then on the exhale slowly lift the feet about a foot off the ground. Inhale and lower.

An alternative is to raise the feet and then hold them in place. Use burst breathing as you hold, then lower slowly, Try to keep the body as relaxed as possible.

SIT UPS

CIRCLE UPS

This exercise uses the momentum of a rolling movement to perform a sit up. This makes it less strain on the back and abs and is also a good foundation exercise for learning to fall and roll.

We start the exercise in a sitting position, with the back nice and straight. Keep the legs relaxed throughout the movement.

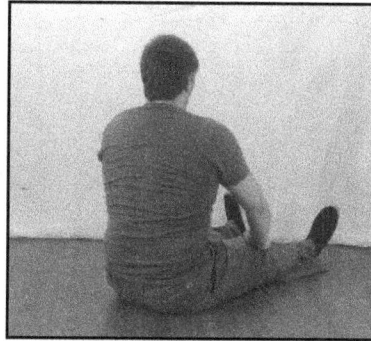

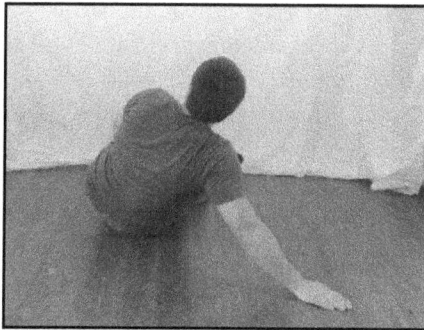

Allow the body to fall to the right and slightly back. The hand can contact the floor, but be sure not to brace the arm.

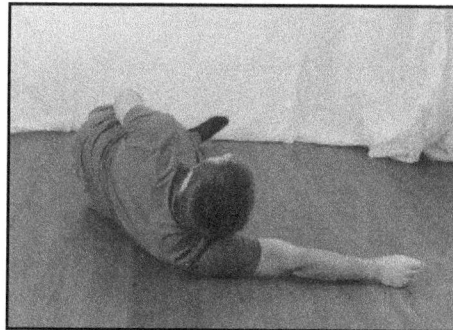

Instead, allow the hand to slide away from you, so bringing the side of the body smoothly to the floor.

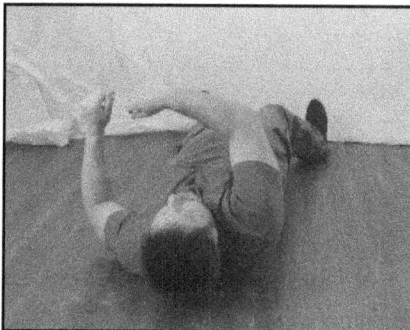

Now roll across the shoulders, you can use a slight rotation to help, exactly the same as our earlier Joint Rotation exercise.

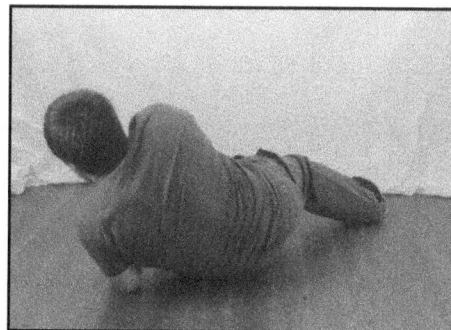

Come onto the left hand side and use a little support from the left arm to continue the roll into an upward movement.

SIT UPS

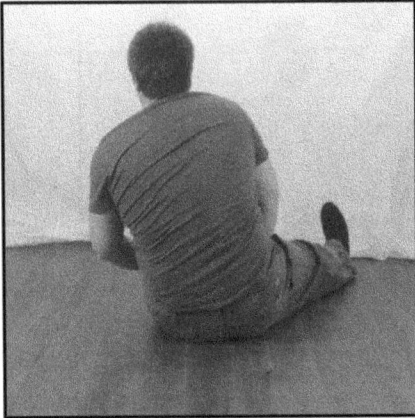

The momentum takes the body up and you return to the start position. Repeat in the same direction a few times, then fall to the left.

Another option is alternate falling right, then left and so on. Whichever way you, get used to exhaling on the fall and roll, inhaling on the lift.

FULL SIT UP

The full sit up is simple, though remember our earlier caution about back issues. Start position is to lay flat on the floor. Keep the body and particularly the legs as relaxed as possible. You may find at first that tension in the legs makes you lift the feet in order to bring the body upright. Instead, we need to be activating the core muscles to perform the movement.

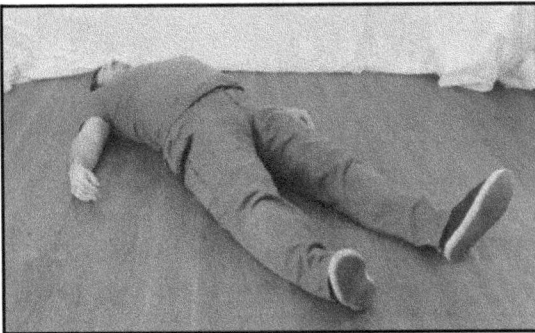

Inhale, then exhale and sit the body straight up. The spine should remain straight all the way through the movement, do not slouch. Keep the arms at the side, again in order to engage the core fully. Inhale and sit back.

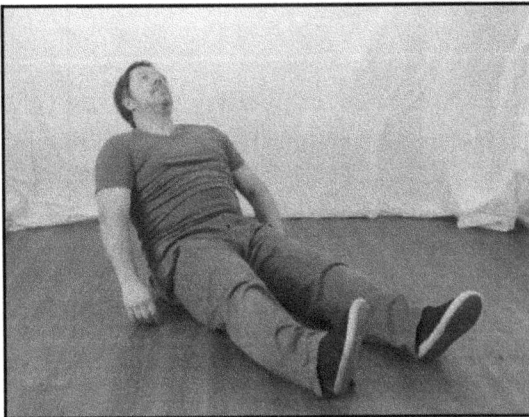

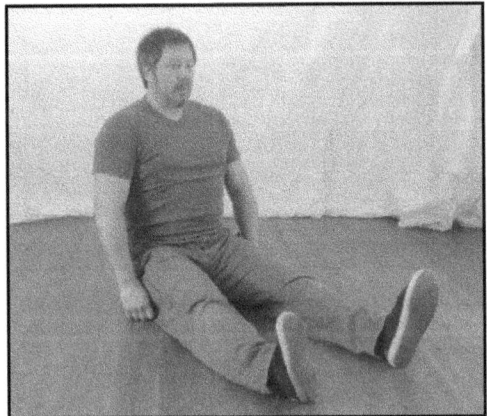

SIT UPS

STATIC SIT UP

This is the sit up version of the plank. From the start position, bring the body up to an angle of around 45 degrees. Maintain this position for while, say a count of ten to begin with. Then, slowly lower back down again. When static, keep the breathing working - you may wish to burst breath to help the body stay relaxed. You can also experiment with holding the body at greater or lesser angles.

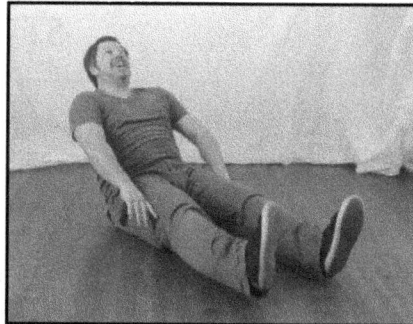

LEG RAISE

Our final version of the sit up is the leg raise. I will again add a note of caution in here for anyone with back or neck issues. Also, if you are not used to this type of movement I would advise getting good at the basic sit ups before trying the leg raise. The key, as always, is to work step by step, establishing your comfortable range of motion to start with.

From a prone position, inhale. Then, as you exhale lift the feet directly up and over the head. If you find this tough at first, you can try starting from a sitting position and letting the body fall softly back. As you do so, use the momentum of the fall to lift your legs.

Bring the feet over as far as you can. In time, you may be able to bring the toes right down to the ground. The bodyweight should rest on the shoulders, not the neck! See how the hands can also help with support.

From here, inhale and return to the start position.

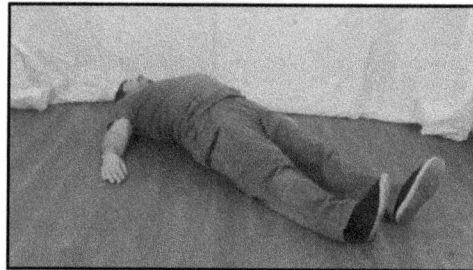

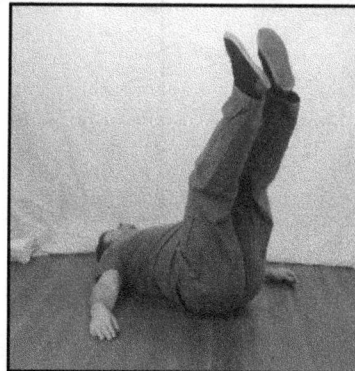

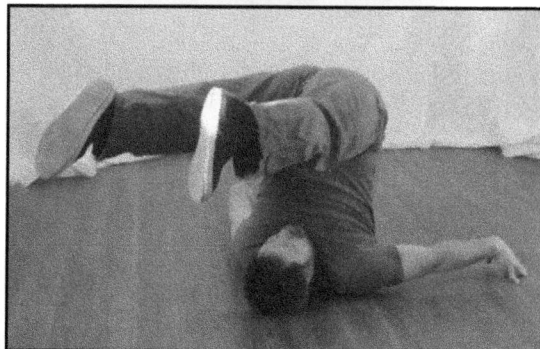

CHAPTER FIVE

STRETCHING

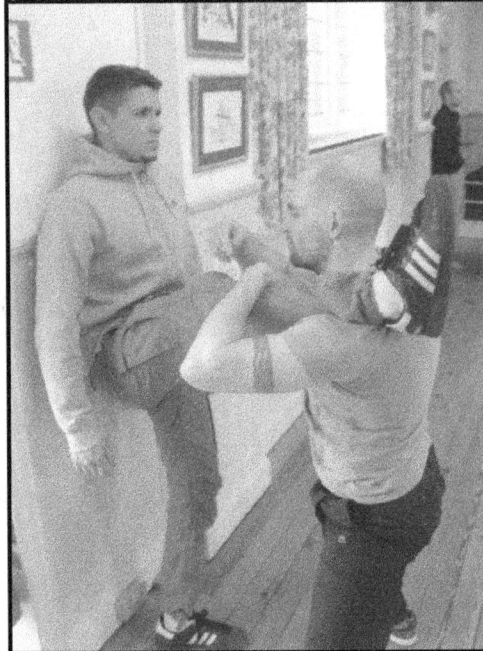

STRETCHING

Stretching is a very natural activity, it's often the first thing we do on waking up in the morning. Animals stretch frequently and quite naturally, people should do the same!

Unfortunately, people often equate stretching with extreme flexibility, sometimes thinking that ligaments and tendons can be stretched. In fact a ligament will only stretch by 6% before it tears and tendons are similar. Over-working tendons and ligaments can also result in loss of stability around a joint. For these reasons we avoid ballistic stretching.

Instead, we work slow moving, static and the rather grandly titled Proprioceptive Neuromuscular Facilitation (PNF) methods. As with everything else, we fully incorporate the Four Pillars into our stretching, to ensure our stretches are not only effective but safe as well. So let us explain the procedure for each type of stretch.

SLOW MOVING STRETCH

This is the type of everyday stretch we do, such as when yawning. First inhale, then perform the stretch on the exhale. The key is to keep the muscle relaxed. Inhale and return to the original position.

STATIC STRETCH

The same as above, but rather than return to the start position, we hold the stretch for a period of time. Around 30 seconds is okay to start. Once again, keep the muscles relaxed. Sometimes it helps to hold the stretched limb in place. If the muscle feels particularly tense, you can use burst breathing to help relax it. In any case, do not hold the breath while you hold the stretch!

RUSSIAN STRETCH

I know the PNF method as the Russian Stretch, as it is the main method used in Systema. This method aims to overcome the stretch reflex. This is where a muscle that is moved beyond its usual ROM tenses up in order to protect the body.

Now this is fine in some situations but problems arise when our ROM becomes restricted, due to lack of use, poor posture and so on. Our own muscle then tries to prevent us working to our full, natural ROM. Think of it as a fear response, how people tense in a stressful situation, also called the Freeze Response.

Fortunately, we can overcome this response in order to fully regain our natural movement capabilities. This is why my Russian teacher, who at the age of almost 60 still moves like a cat, often says "I am not flexible, I am free."

We work from a static stretch position, with the muscle at maximum stretch. As you reach that point you will feel the muscle tighten, that's the stretch reflex kicking in. In order to overcome it, inhale and tense that particular muscle even more. Tense it as much

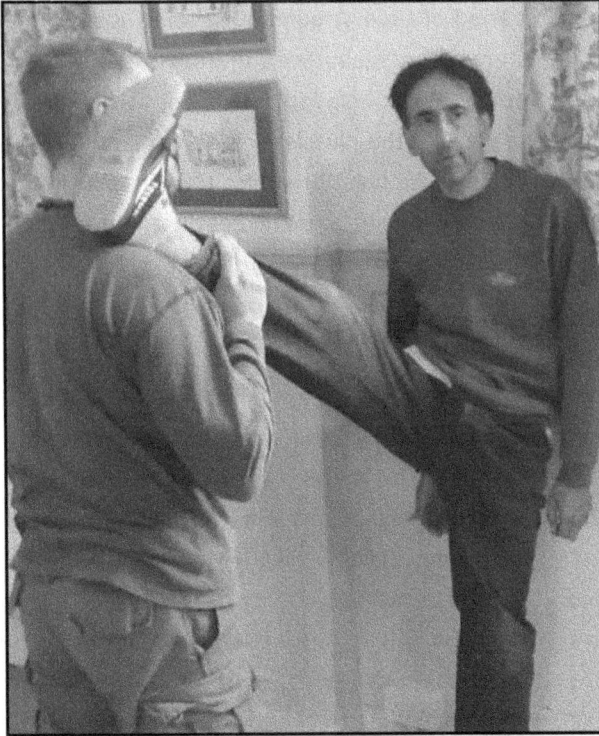

great little exercise for releasing tension in general. Applied to stretching, it helps us regain our full ROM.

Of course, there is a point beyond which muscles will not stretch, but you will be surprised how far you can go over time. Also this method should be pain free, if you feel any sudden or sharp pain then come out of the stretch straight away. Incidentally, when coming out of any static stretch, do so slowly, allow the muscle to settle gently back into its former position.

THE STRETCHES

To start I am going to show you a range of basic stretches for the upper and lower body. When it comes to legs, especially, there are hundreds of stretching exercises and it is not too hard to come up with your own either. The important things to remember are the Four Pillars and to work slowly and steadily.

In terms of routine, I suggest you begin by following the "three and hold" method. This means we do each movement as a slow stretch three times, followed by a static stretch. This will give us a good overall stretch routine, plus help highlight any areas that may need more work. You can then go back to those problem areas and work the Russian Stretch to get in little deeper. Remember to work both sides!

as you can and hold both the breath and the tension for at least thirty seconds. Then exhale and release the tension. You should find that you can now get more movement from the muscle, up until the next point of tension.

So we are literally trying to overload the muscle with tension, so forcing it to relax. This is also one reason we tend to work the exhale-relax cycle, we are conditioning the muscles to subconsciously relax on every exhale.

If you want to practice this without a stretch, simply inhale and tense you arms. Hold for as long as you can, then exhale and release all the tension. You should feel your arms are more relaxed than before you started, it's a

UPPER BODY

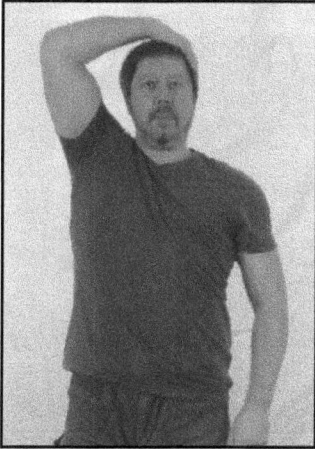

Place the right hand on the left side of the head. Inhale.

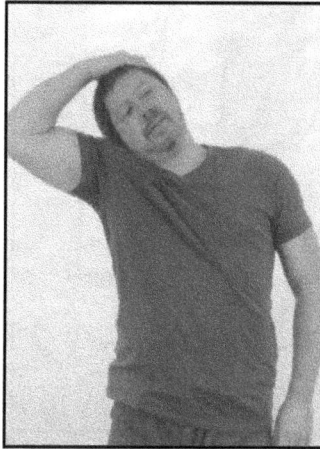

Exhale as you gently pull the head towards the right shoulder.

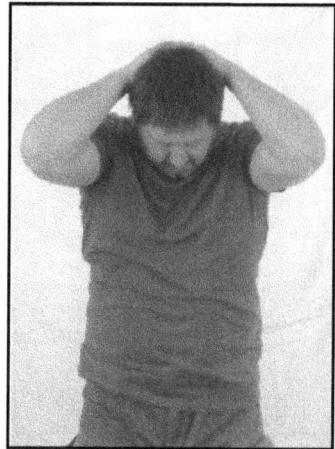

Place the palms on the back of the head. Inhale. Pull the head forward on the exhale

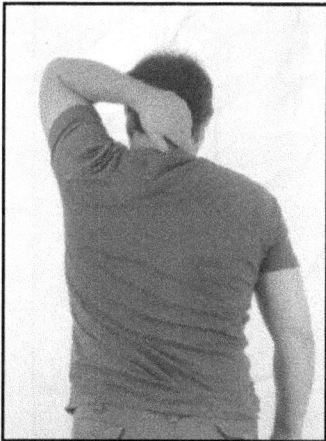

Place the left hand behind the neck. Inhale.

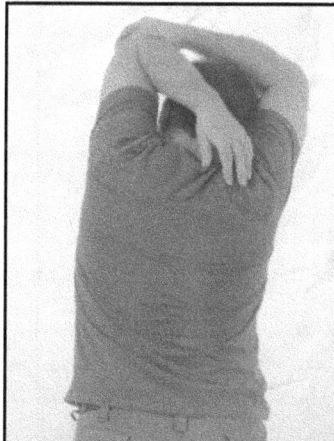

Grab the elbow with the right hand. Exhale and gently pull the left elbow to the right.

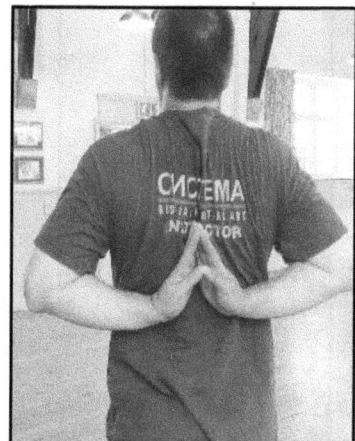

Touch the fingertips together behind the back, inhale. Exhale and push the fingers up as high as you can, try and get the palms to touch.

UPPER BODY

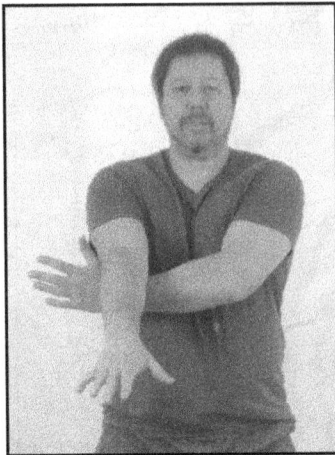

Place the left hand under the right elbow. Inhale.

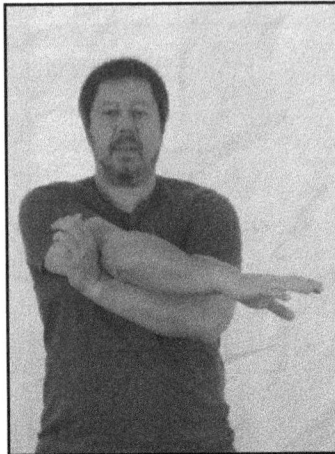

Exhale as you pull the right arm across the body.

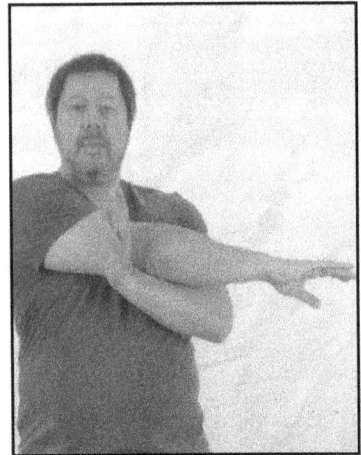

As you pull the arm relax the back and allow the shoulder blades to open.

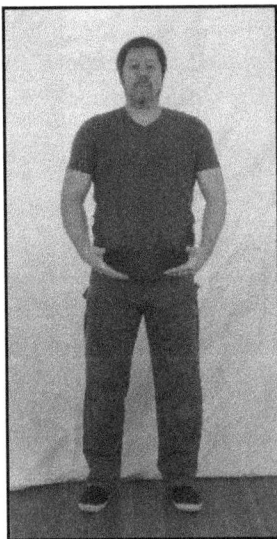

Begin with arms at the waist, palms up. Inhale.

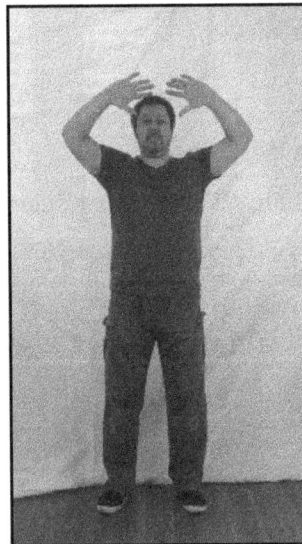

Exhale as you rotate the palms outwards and begin to raise them.

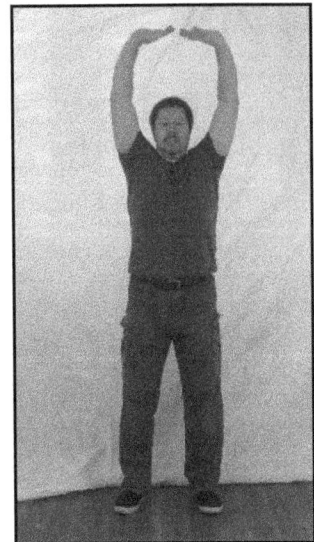

Push the palms up as high as you can but be sure to keep the shoulder relaxed. Inhale as you circle the hands back to the waist.

UPPER BODY

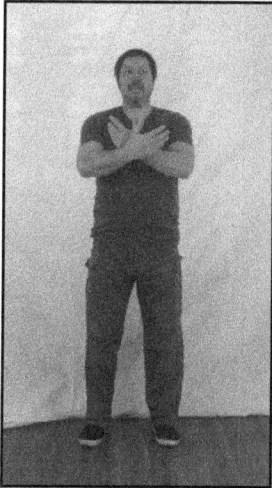

Cross the hands in front
of the chest, right hand
outside. Inhale.

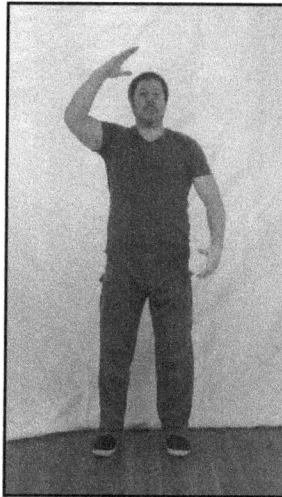

Exhale as you rotate the
right palm up, the left
hand moves down/

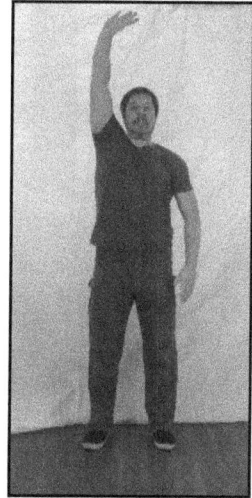

Push the hands up and
down. Inhale as the
hands cross, repeat on
the other side.

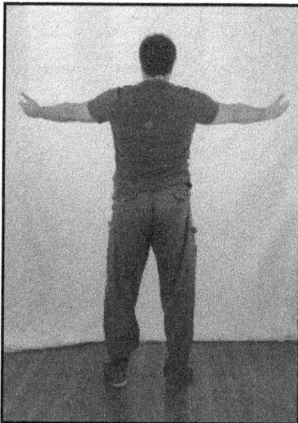

Hold the hands out to
the side.
Inhale.

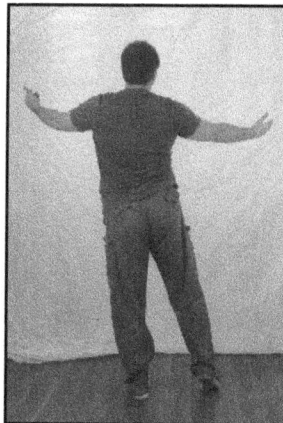

Shift the weight into
the left foot and raise
the right heel.

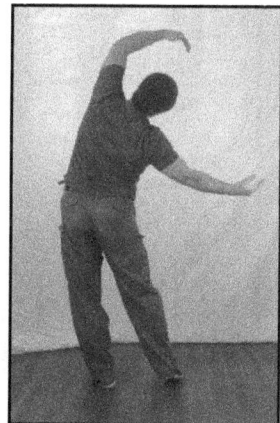

Exhale as you bend to
the side, pointing the
left fingers towards the
right palm.

WAIST

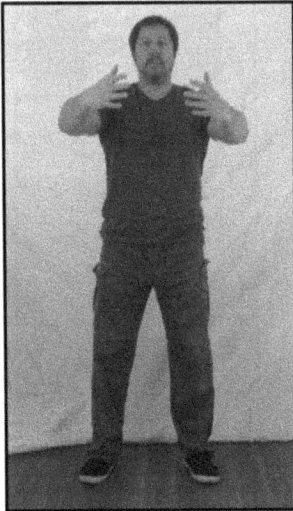

Hold the hands in front of you at chest height, palms turned in. Inhale.

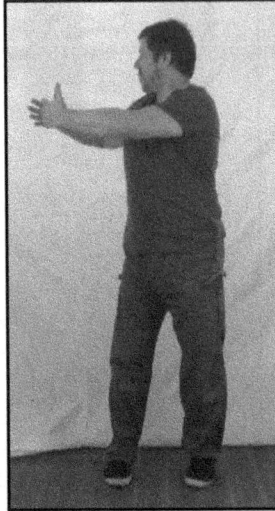

Rotate the body to the side, turning the waist as far as you can.

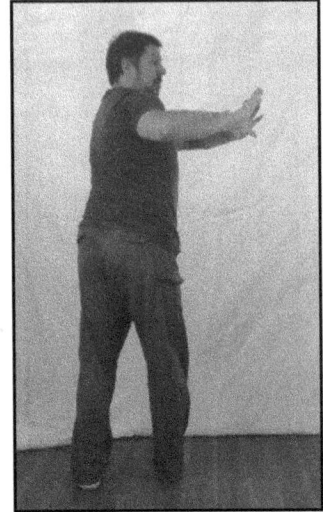

Exhale as you turn the palms outwards and push. Allow the shoulder blades to open.

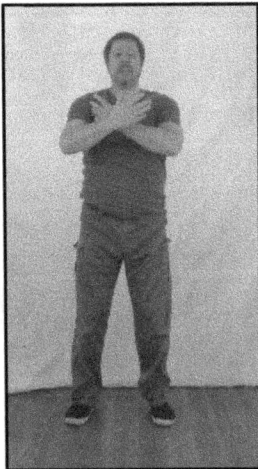

Cross the hands in front of the chest
Inhale.

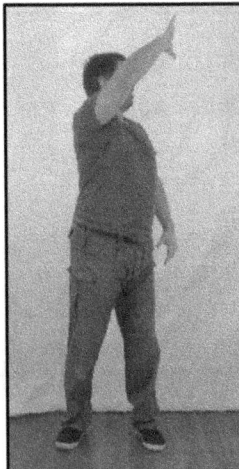

Push right hand up and left hand down and turn at the waist.
Exhale.

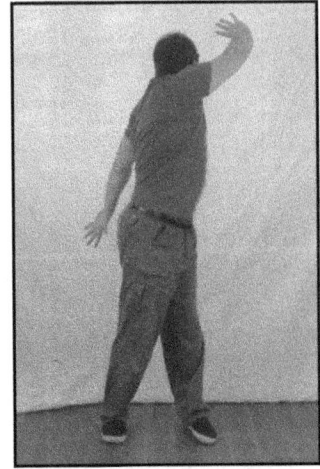

Twist the waist as far as you can while pushing up and down with the hands.

WAIST

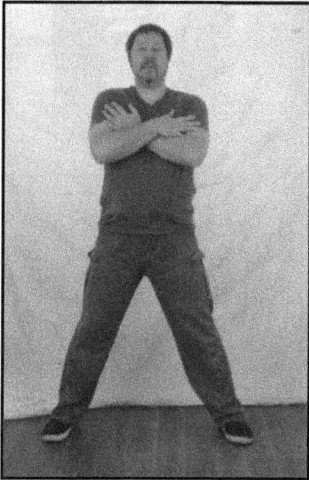

Cross the arms over
your chest.
Inhale.

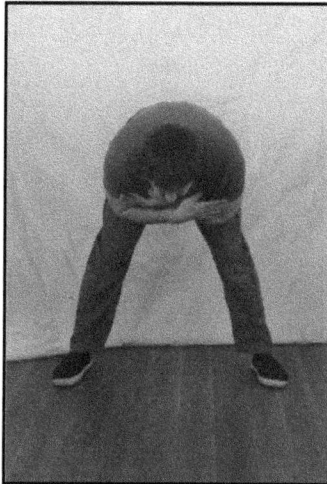

Exhale as you bend forward.
Just go as far a comfortable
and do not slouch. Lead the
up and down movement with
the head.

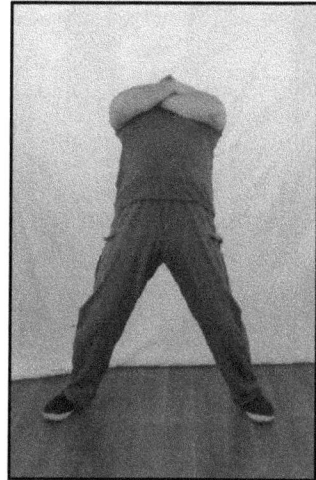

From the same start
position, exhale and bend
back. Again, do not force the
movement.

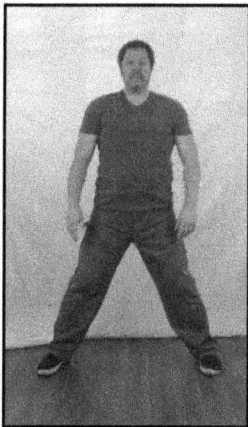

Stand in a wide stance,
with the feet just over
shoulder width apart.
Inhale.

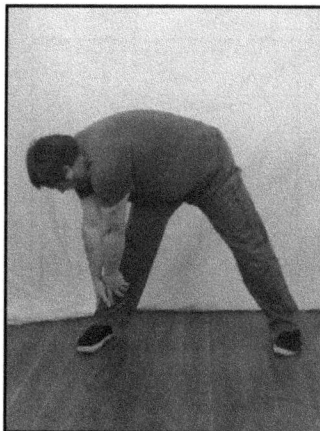

Exhale as you bend at
the waist. Reach down
and grab the right leg.

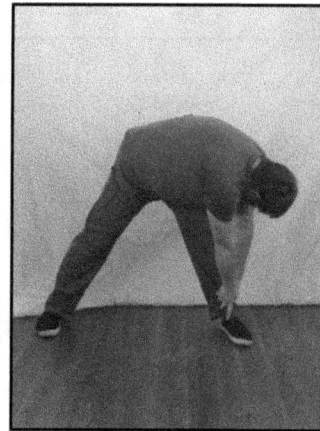

Inhale and return to
start position, then
repeat on the left.
Again, lead with the
head.

LEGS

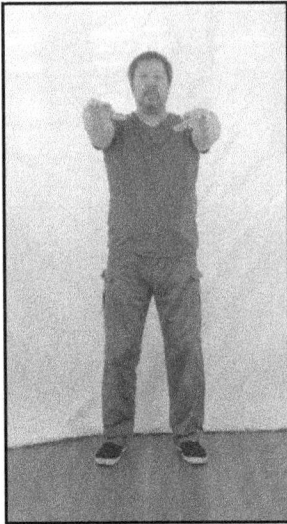

Stand with feet at shoulder width, raise the hands to shoulder height. Inhale.

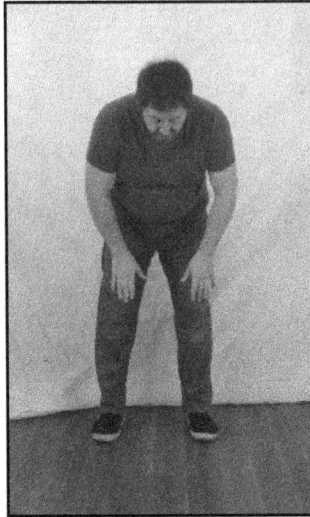

Exhale as you bend at the waist.

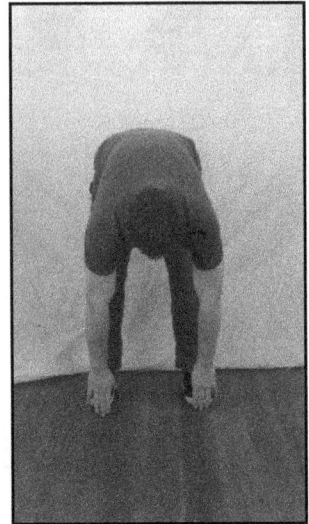

Reach down as far as you can, stretching out the lower back. Lead with the head.

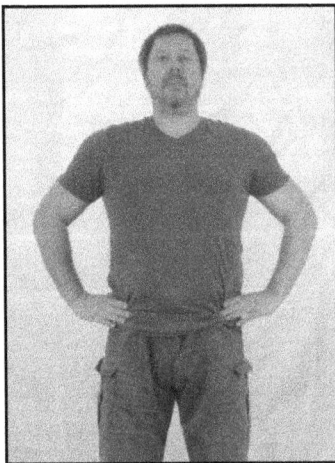

Bring the feet to shoulder width, place hands on hips. Inhale.

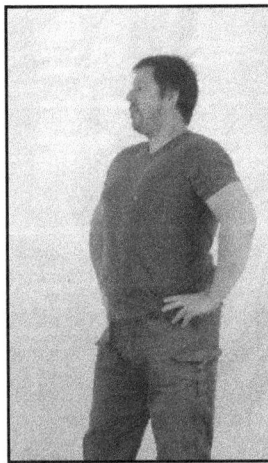

Place weight in the left leg, turn to the right and lift the right toes.

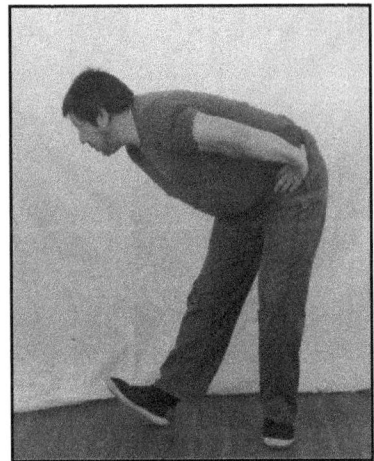

Exhale as you bend forward, to your comfortable ROM. Lead with the head again, stretching the lower back out.

LEGS

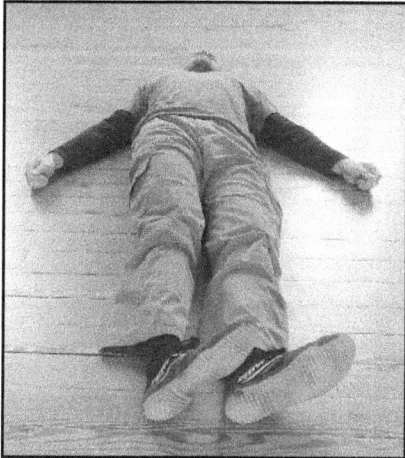

Lay on your back, feet upright, inhale. Exhale as you pull the toes back towards you. Inhale and relax. Next, exhale as you move the feet to each side, inhale as they return to upright position.

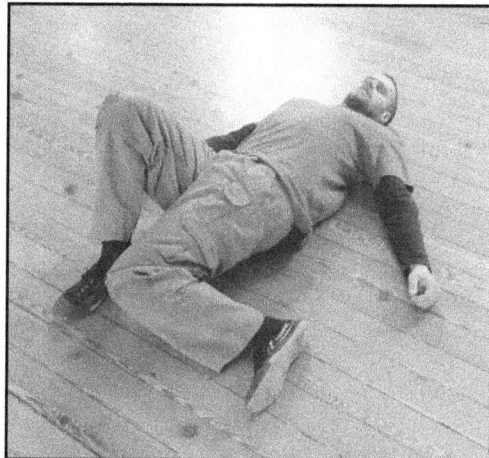

Bring the feet in, raising up the knees. Inhale.
As you exhale, move one knee down towards the opposite ankle. Inhale and return to the start position. Try and keep the hips in contact with the floor throughout.

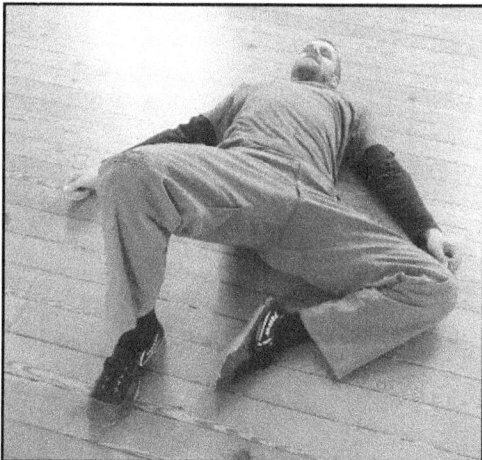

Repeat the last exercise, but this time the knee goes down to the outside.

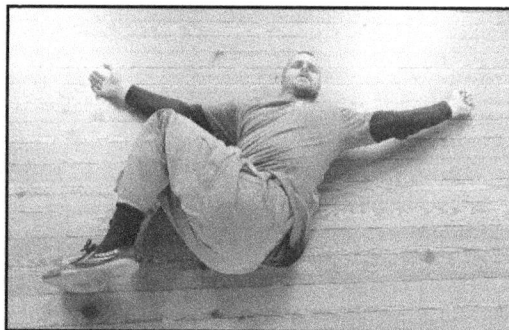

Bring the knees up a little higher, so that the feet are off the ground. Take the arms out to the sides. Inhale.
As you exhale, take both knees across to the side and down. Inhale and return to the start position.

LEGS

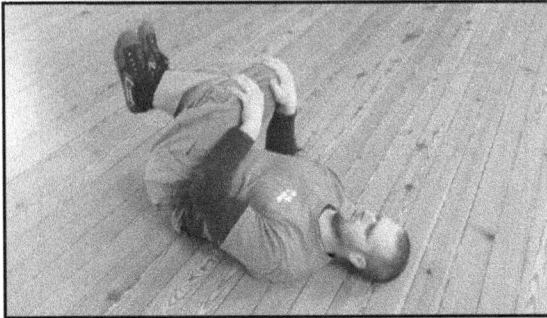

Keeping the feet off of the ground, place
the hands over the knees.
Make circles with the knees, from
small to large, then back again.
Repeat in the opposite direction.
Keep the breathing natural throughout.

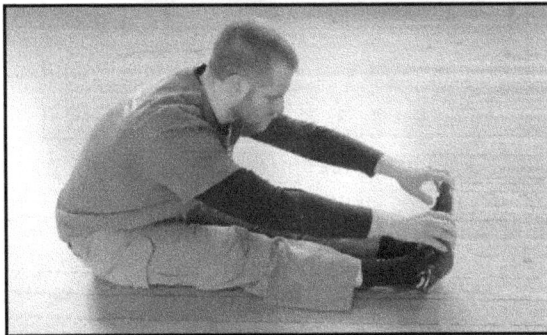

Sit up with your legs stretched out in front
of you. Inhale.
Exhale as you lean forward to touch your
toes. Try and keep the back straight, do not
slouch. If you cannot reach the toes at first,
just go as far as you can.
If you can reach the toes, you can also pull
them back to increase the stretch.

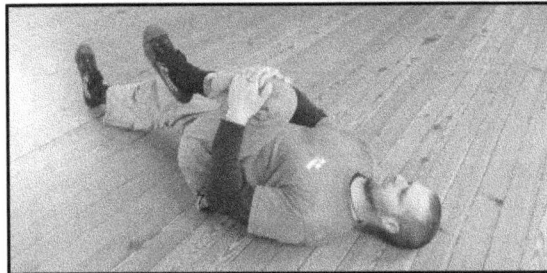

Lay back and raise one leg. Grasp the knee
with both hands. Inhale.
Exhale as you pull the knee up towards the
chest. Make sure you keep the direction
of the pull straight, do not pull out
to the side.

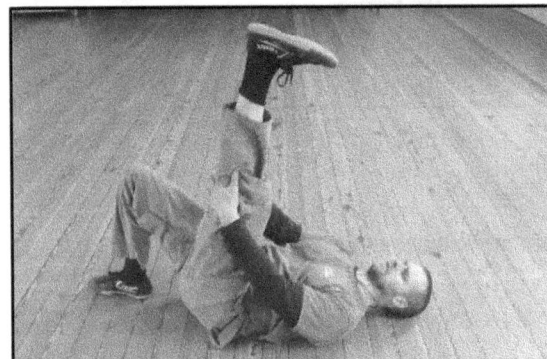

Lift the leg up and place both hands
behind the knee. Inhale.
Exhale as you straighten the leg and
pull the knee towards the chest.

LEGS

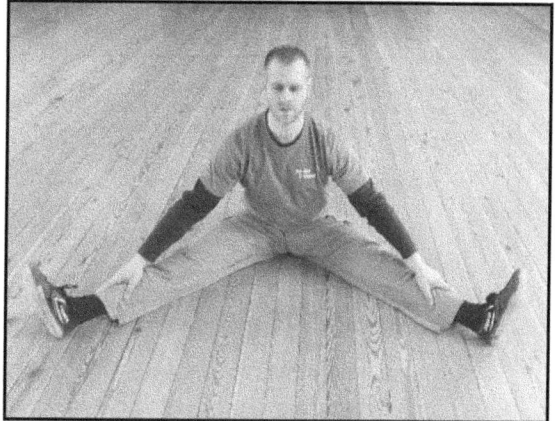

Place the feet flat on the floor, knees raised.
Now take one ankle and place it on the
opposite knee. Inhale.
As you exhale, slowly push the
knee away from you.
Inhale and release the pressure.

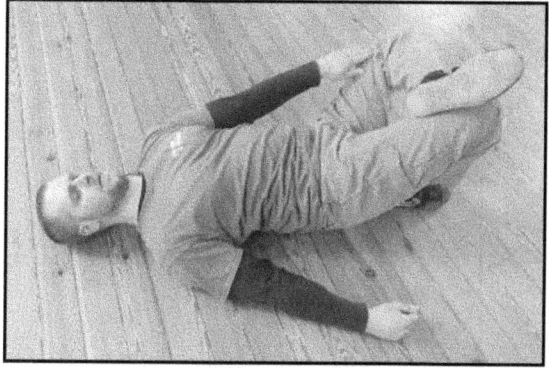

Sit upright and bring both legs out at an
angle. Inhale.
Exhale and take your hands out to rest on
the shins. Keep the back straight.

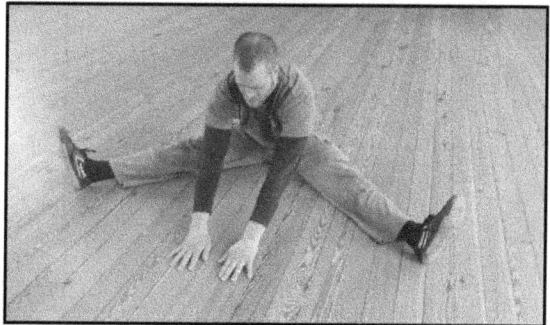

From the same start position, exhale as
you lean forward. Try and place the
palms flat on the floor.
It is important again to keep the back
straight. Slouching means the body gets
lower, but you are not stretching so much!

LEGS

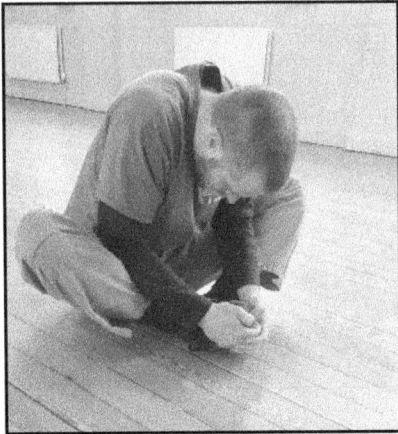

Sitting upright, grab the feet and pull
them in together. If you can, bring
the feet sole to sole. Inhale.
As you exhale, lean forward and at the same
time try and push the knees down.
Inhale and return to upright position.

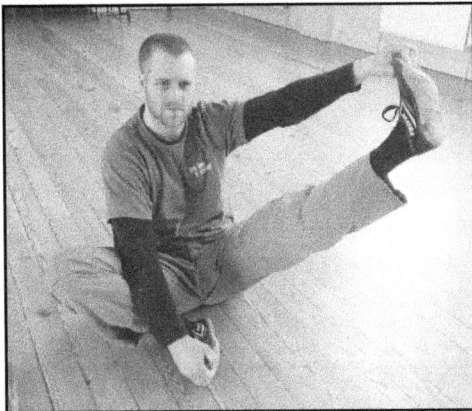

From the last position, grab the feet
separately. Inhale.
As you exhale, straighten one leg out,
keeping a firm grasp of the toes.
Inhale and return to the start position.

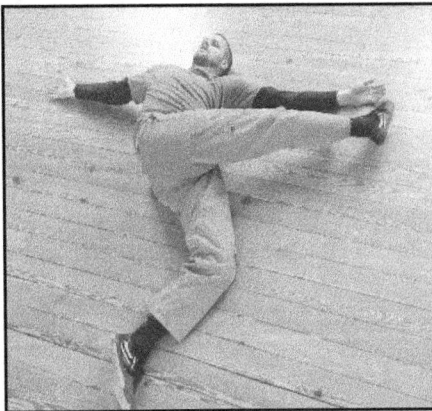

Lay back, with arms out to the sides. Inhale.
As you exhale, take one foot towards
the opposite hand. If you can reach far
enough, you can grab the toes to hold
the leg in place.
Try and keep the shoulders in contact
with the floor throughout.

LEGS

Stretch one leg out in front and fold the
other back. You can use the hands to
support your weight. Inhale.
Exhale and lean the body forward, you can
reach for the toes as before.
Once again, be sure not to slouch.

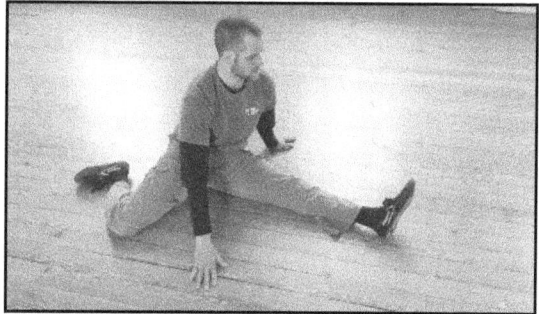

From the above position, bend the lead
leg so that the sole of the foot rests
against the rear thigh.
This is a very good resting position and, like
the Cossack Squat, you should try spending
some time in it each day.
Be sure to maintain a straight spine.

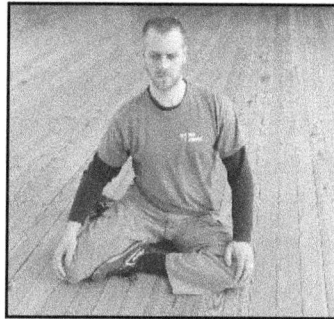

To stretch from this position, inhale. Then
exhale as you raise the arm and lean back.
You can support the body weight on your
elbow as shown.
Inhale and return to upright position.

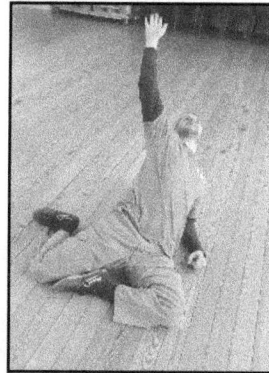

You can try the same thing but leaning in
different directions. Here, you can see
how to bring the palms to the floor
to get a good stretch for hips and lower
back.

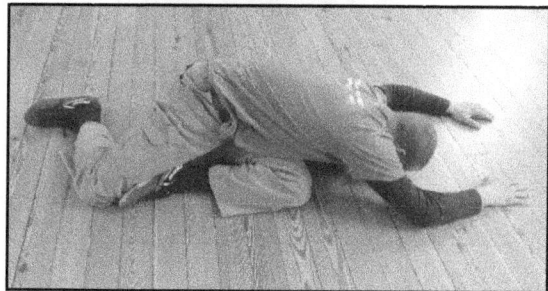

PARTNER STRETCHES

Solo stretching is a very good habit to get into and will certainly help with health and mobility. However, sometimes there is only so far you can go with a solo stretch.

This is where partner stretching comes into its own. A partner can help you push beyond your solo range of motion, can provide support for some exercises and can also twist you in interesting ways!

Of course, all the same principles and procedures apply as with the solo work. When working solo we are obviously aware of our own body. When stretching with a partner we must exercise that same sensitivity to our partner. Listen to their breathing, watch and feel for signs of discomfort and tension. Never rush your partner and never, ever move them quickly while under tension. At the end of each stretch allow the body to move slowly back to its neutral position.

From the other perspective, give your assistant feedback, tell them if you need less or more of a push. If you feel any sharp pain or discomfort tell your partner to stop immediately. Remember to work with your breathing, never try and muscle through a stretch. Above all, take your time and work in small increments. Better to think long tem gain than short term glory.

Almost every part of the body can be stretched and the exercises here are by no means exhaustive, but they will give you a good start, as well as a base to create your own ideas. Once you have the basics down, be creative!

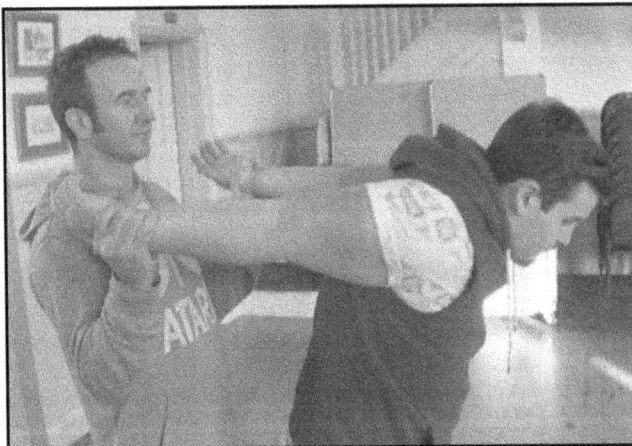

Take your partners wrists and, keeping the hands at shoulder width or wider, slowly lift. Hold in position as your partner relaxes their shoulders.
Then slowly move the hands in towards each other. When tension comes back into the shoulders, stop the movement and run through the Russian Stretching procedure. You should then be able to move the hands a little closer.
When done, release the hands slowly.

PARTNER STRETCHES

You can work the same exercise with the person laying face down on the floor. The head is turned to one side and the hands are again held out at shoulder width. Move the hands slowly together in the same way, pausing for the tense/relax cycle where necessary.
When finished, lower the arms slowly to the floor.
These exercises can be challenging if you have tense shoulders,so please practice them with care.

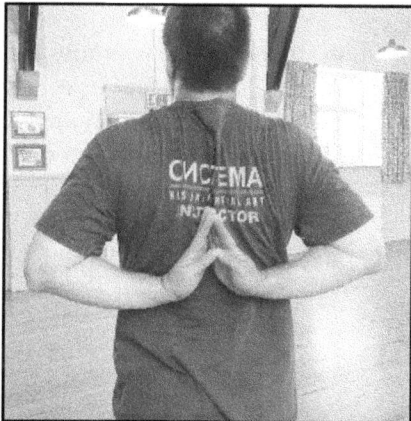

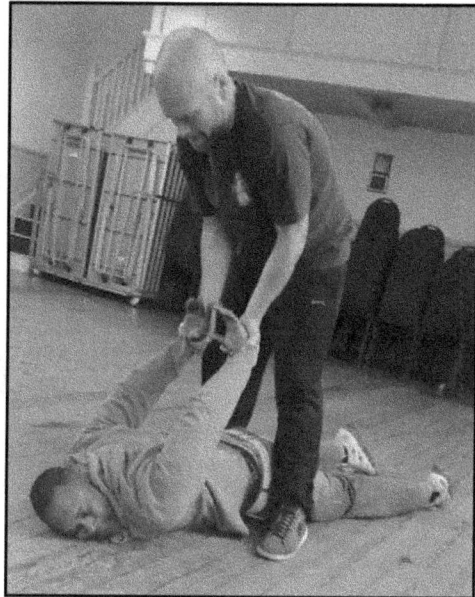

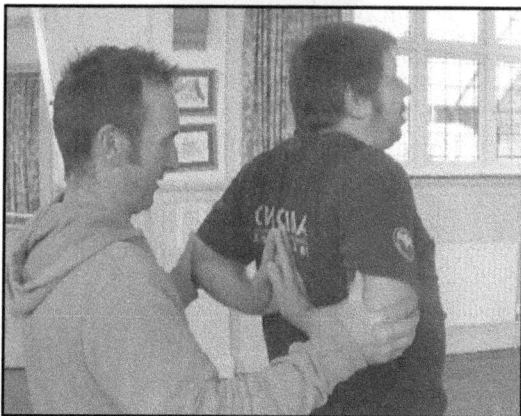

There is also a two person version of the hands behind the back exercise. Start the same way, touch the fingertips together, then push upwards to bring the palms towards each other. Once you stop, your partner holds your elbows. You inhale, then exhale as your partner slowly and gently pulls your elbows back.

Hold the position and burst breathe. Allow the chest to open and the shoulders to move back a little. Once done, your partner slowly releases the elbows and helps lower the hands if required.

PARTNER STRETCHES

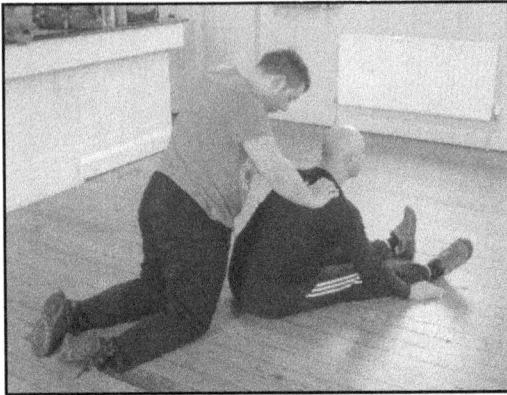

Sit up straight with your legs out in front. Inhale. Exhale as you lean forward and reach for your toes. Your partner gently pushes you forward. Once again, you can work as a moving push and/or hold in a static position with burst breathing.

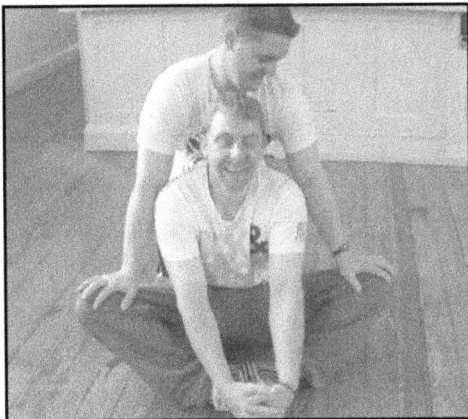

Sit up straight, grasp your toes and pull the soles of the feet together. As you exhale, your partner applies gentle downward pressure on your thighs. Follow the usual protocols and release slowly when finished.

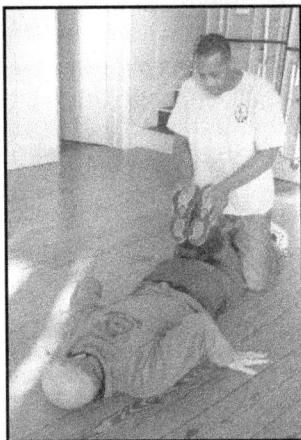

Lay on your front, arms at your side. Your partner holds your feet and slowly moves them towards your backside. Exhale. Hold the position and burst breath, try and let the thighs relax as much as possible. Once again, release slowly when finished.

PARTNER STRETCHES

Sit up straight with legs out to the sides. Your partner takes up position as shown, with their feet against your lower legs. Your partner then clasps your hands as you lean forward.
The partner can pull a little on your arms to assist, while pushing out a little from the feet. This is a great exercise to work the Russian Stretch with.

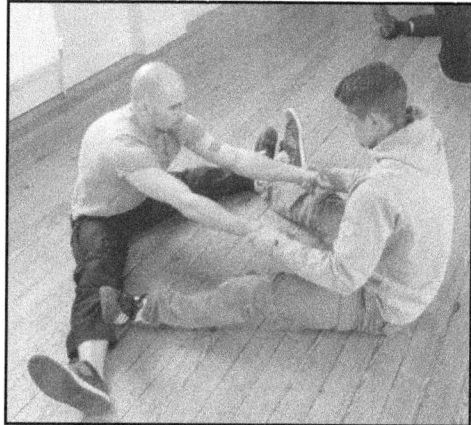

Stand with your back to the wall. Try and keep the back in contact with the wall throughout the exercise.
Your partner squats down and you place your ankle on their shoulder.
Keeping good posture, your partner now slowly stands up, raising your foot.
If the leg begins to tense, have your partner stop and run through the Russian Stretch method.
When finished, bend your knee and place the sole of the foot on your partners chest.
Now slowly push them away and allow the foot to go back to the floor.

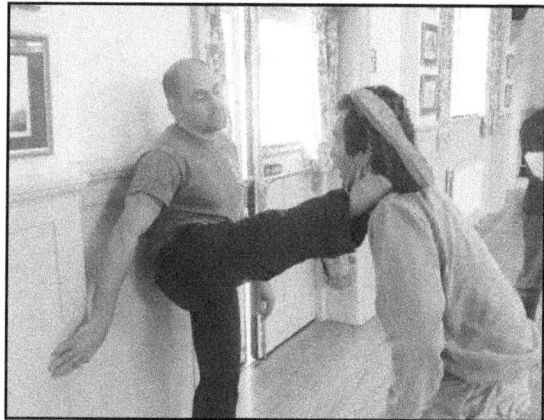

Another method of stretching is to have your partner take a leg or arm and gently twist it in various directions.
If you find an area of particular tension, ask your partner to hold that position as you breathe and relax.

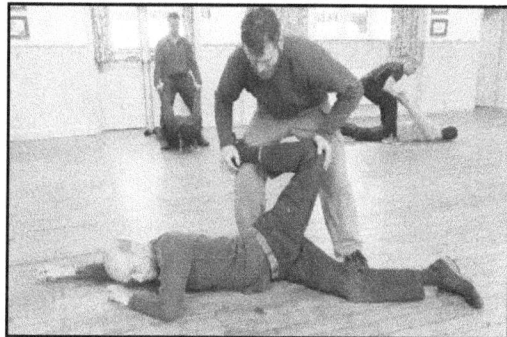

CHAPTER SIX

STICK WORK

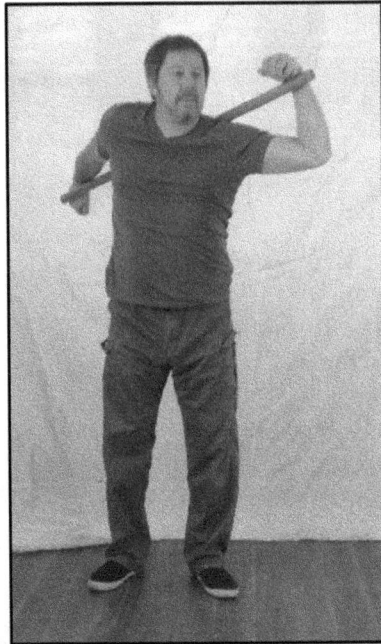

THE STICK

Using equipment is very common in modern fitness training, especially if you are gym user. However, the use of training equipment goes back as far as you care to look. Everything from rocks and logs have been used, along with weapons, tools like sledgehammers and more specialised equipment such as kettle bells.

There are pros and cons to using anything, but I feel that the older types of equipment training have more pros than cons. They are easy to find, generally cheap, or even free, and adaptable to many types of exercise. In terms of weight training, they are also free weights. Certain equipment exercises also work ROM and encourage good posture and movement. So using equipment can be very useful for our type of training.

One of the simplest and most useful piece of equipment is the humble stick. We can use it for stretching, mobility, strength and posture training. You can do a lot of exercises with a broomstick but I recommend you get something stronger for the weight bearing exercises. I use a curtain pole from a hardware shop cut down to about four feet in length. These are a good weight too and sit nicely in the grip.

The first thing to do once you get your stick is simply to handle it. Pass the stick from hand to hand, move around with it a little, get used to the balance and weight.

Remember to always check your surroundings before working with the stick. Not only what is around you but what is above you too! I usually work outside with the stick, even then I have to be aware of the occasional dog that wants to join in with the fun as I am swinging the stick!

The exercises that follow will give you some nice routines as well as a good foundation for more equipment work in the future. We shall be covering the use of hammers, kettle bells and more advanced stick work in future volumes.

Once again, repeat exercises on both sides where appropriate and work slowly and within your comfort zone to start with.

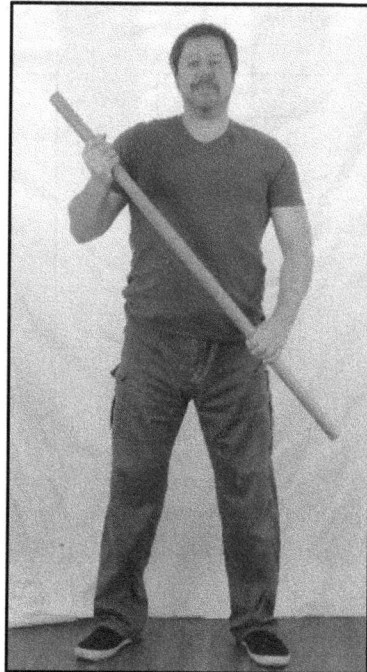

STICK ROTATION

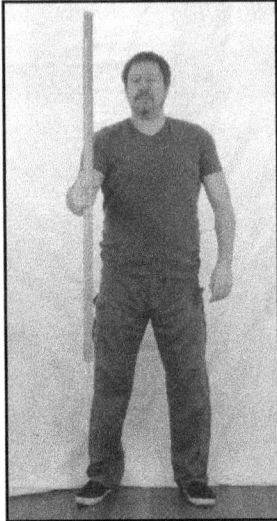

Hold the stick out in front of you in the right hand

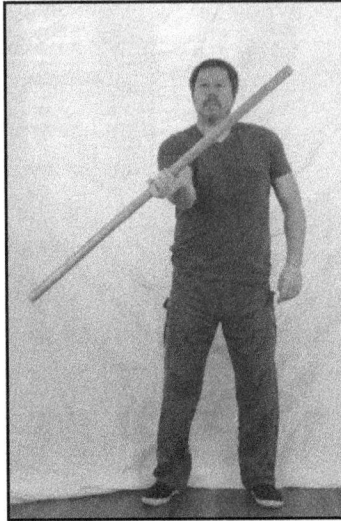

Twist the wrist to rotate the stick left and right.

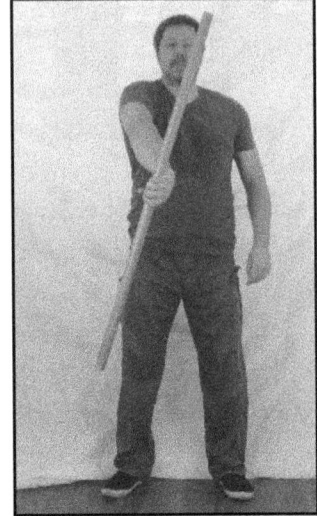

Make sure you keep the shoulder relaxed but maintain a tight grip throughout.

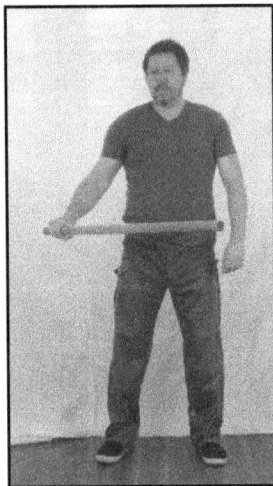

Hold the stick at one end in a tight grip. Throughout this exercise try and keep the stick parallel to the floor.

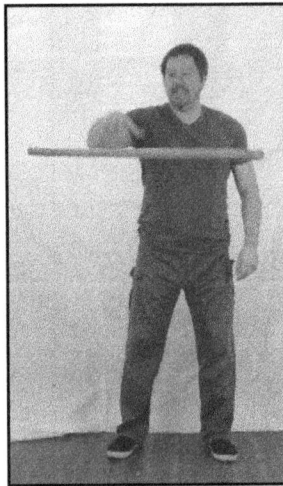

Lift the hand and open the fist to drop the stick.

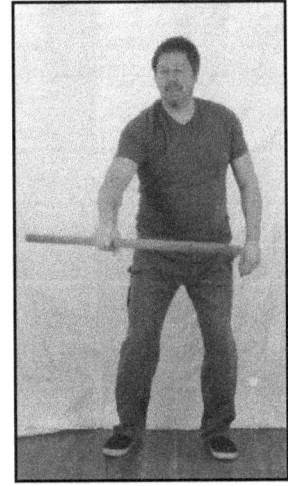

Grab the stick as it falls, with a tight fist. Move your hand along the stick each drop.

STICK ROTATION

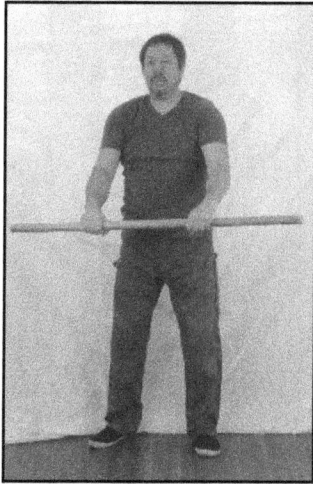

Hold the stick out in front of you in both hands.

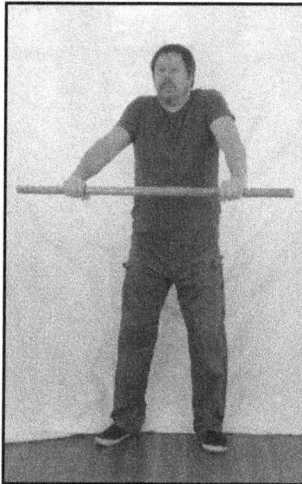

Keeping the stick in place, rotate the shoulders.

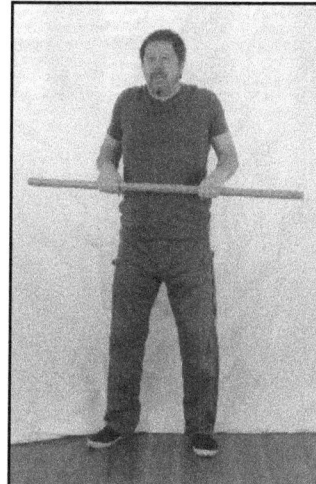

Repeat the same movement with bigger circles, this time you move the stick and shoulders.

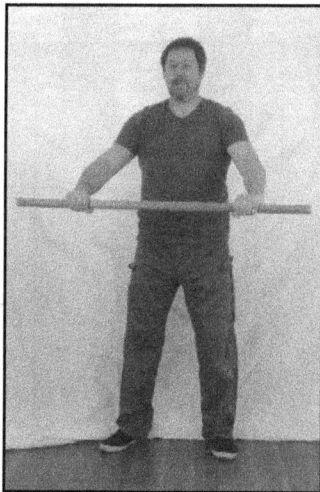

Bring the stick back to the start position.

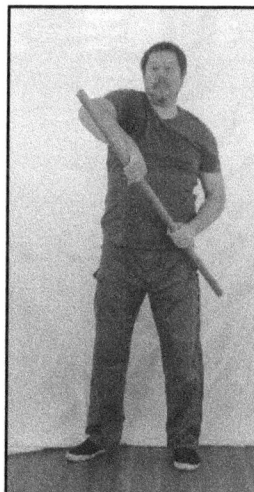

Working from the shoulders, now circle the stick to the sides.

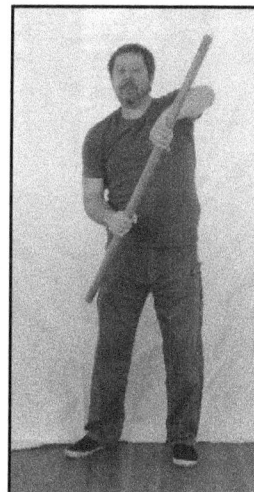

Think of it as a kind of rowing or Figure 8 movement

STICK STRETCHES

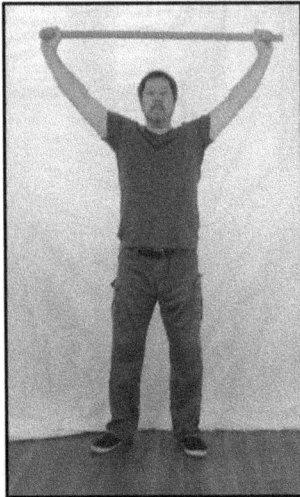

Move the hands to the end of the stick and raise it above your head. Keep the shoulders relaxed.

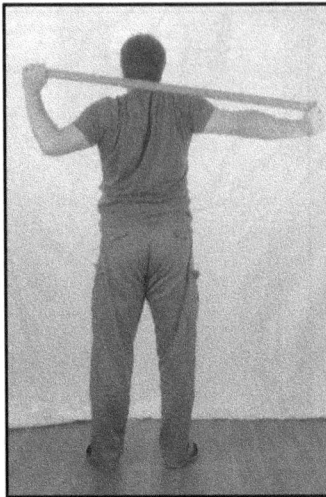

Slowly bring the stick back over the shoulders, keeping them loose.

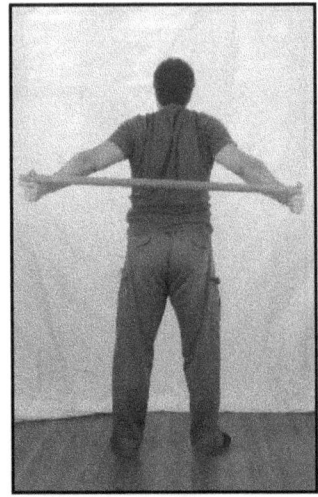

Take the stick as far down as you can. Squeeze the shoulder blades together and hold.

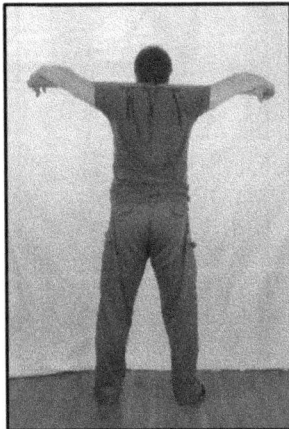

Bring the stick back up and rest it across the shoulders. If you find this difficult, you can hold the stick in the hands instead.

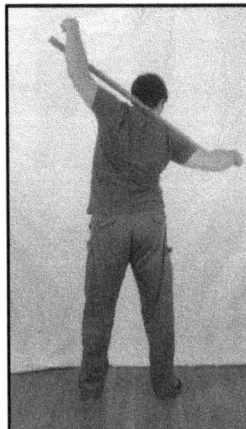

Start making circles with the stick. Think of making a figure 8 pattern again.

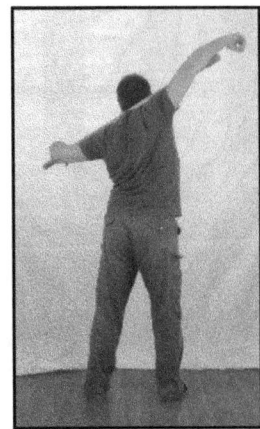

From the same position begin also twisting the torso to the left and right.

STICK STRETCHES

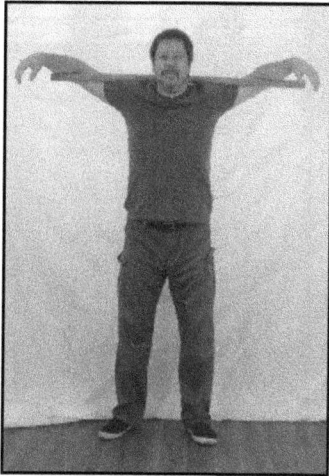

Return the stick to rest over the shoulders.

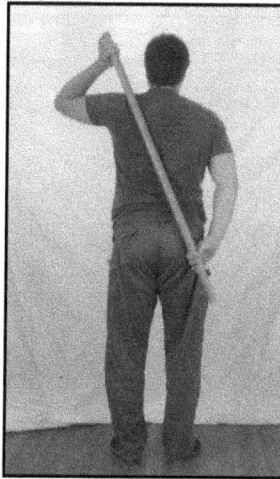

Drop the right end of the stick and grasp it in the right hand

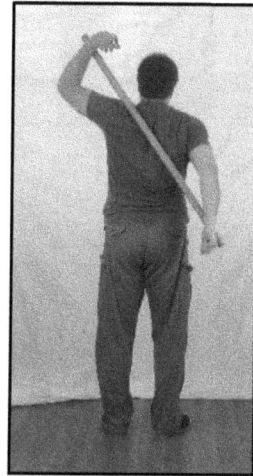

Slide the left hand around the end of the stick, then do the same with the right hand.

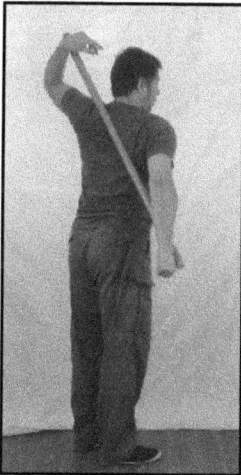

Slowly push the lower end of the stick forward and allow the left shoulder to relax and open.

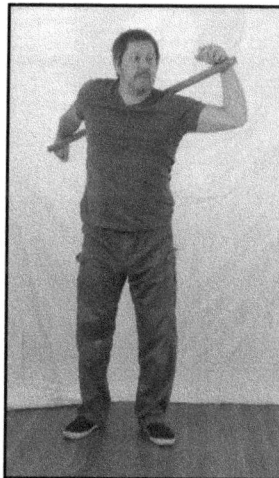

Hold, ease back and repeat. Then push the left hand forward.

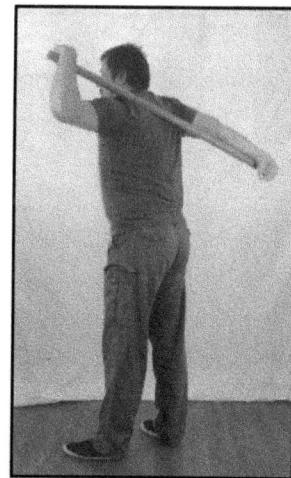

Take a small step forward as you do this and allow the right side to relax

STICK STRENGTH

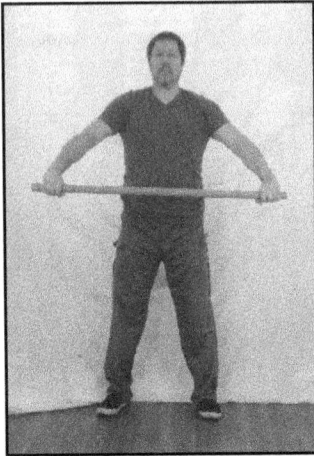

The next exercise uses selective tension. Hold the stick at waist height and grip it tightly to start.

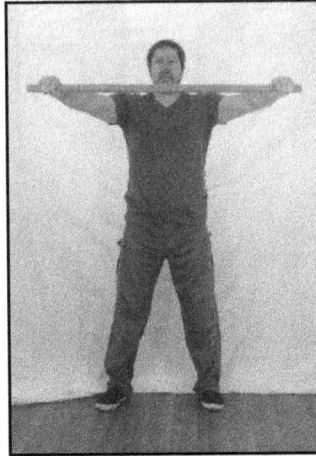

Tense the forearms and pull - imagine you are trying to pull the stick apart. Slowly raise the stick.

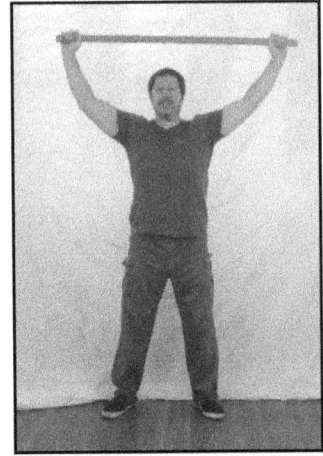

Keeping the tension, lift above the head. Burst breath. Relax at the top, then tense again and lower to start.

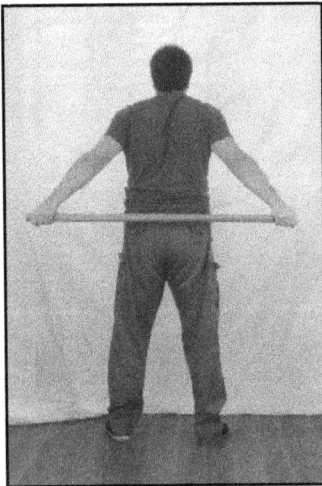

Repeat the same movement but this time pushing in on the stick ends. Then work the same moves with the stick behind you.

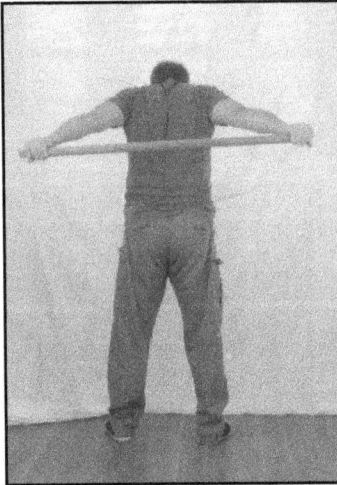

Maintain tension while lifting the hands as high as you can, then lower them down.

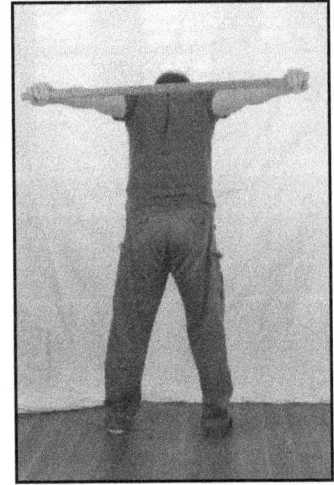

Work once with the pull and once with the push again. Try different grips.

STICK STRENGTH

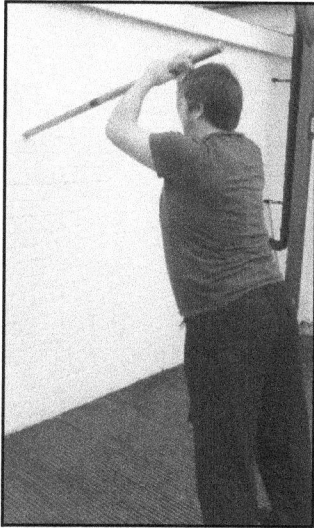

The stick climb is a great upper body exercise. Begin by placing the stick on an incline. At first, you should make sure that the far end is held firmly in place - perhaps leaning into a corner, where the stick cannot slip.

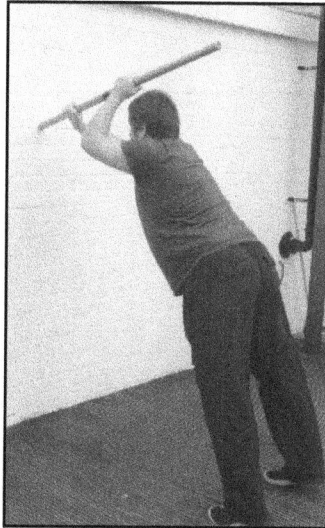

Keep a strong grip and begin "climbing" hand over hand down the stick. Let the heels lift so all your weight is on the stick.

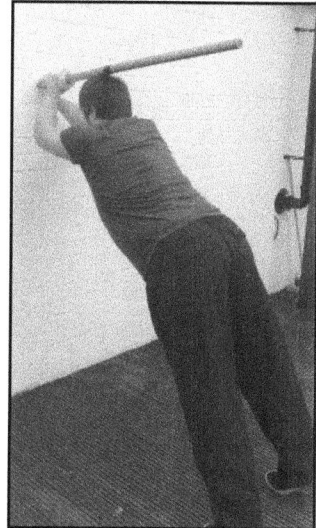

Just go a little way down at first, work up to climbing the full length of the stick. Keep the body as straight as possible. From the end, climb back up to the start point.

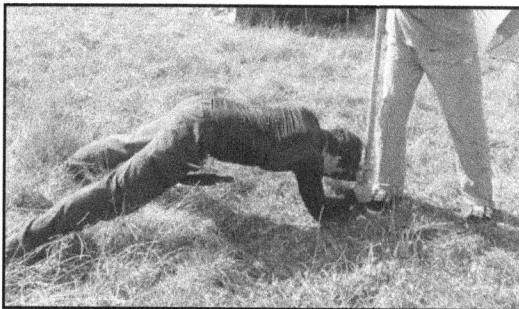

When used to the exercise, you can change the angle of the stick. Get a friend to hold the stick in place for a 90 degree climb. Remember, breathe and keep the body straight.

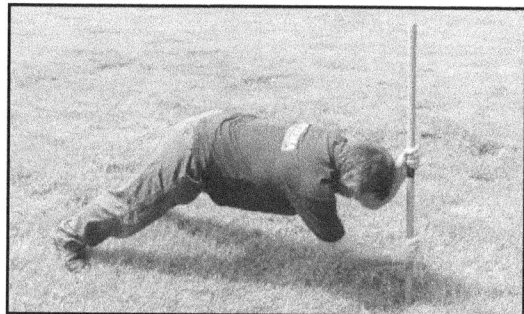

Finally, you can try with an unsupported stick. Work in soft ground and push the stick in a little way. Work both hands together or one hand at a time.

CHAPTER SEVEN

GROUND MOVEMENT

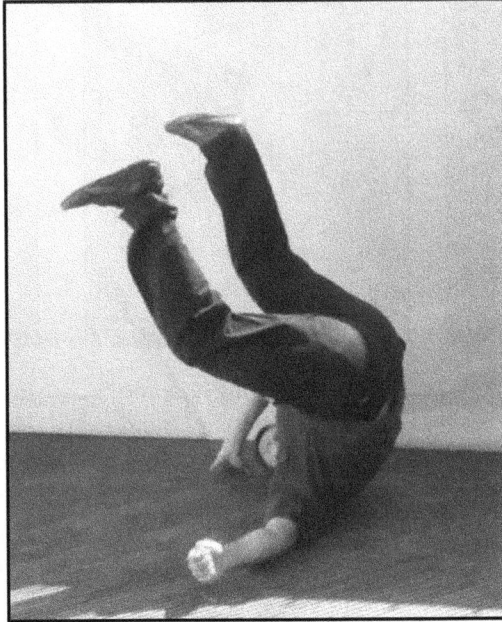

GROUND MOVEMENT

The floor is a very overlooked piece of training equipment. Think about it, it is free, always there and easily accessible! The floor is a great place to develop free movement. For one thing, it offers a lot support so there is little risk of straining ourselves or injury.

As adults, unless you practice martial arts or similar, there is very little interaction with the floor. Even then, I have taught in some martial art sessions where people refused to get on the ground! It is a shame that people have this kind of emotional inhibition and highlights one of the greatest benefits from floor work - rediscovering our capacity for natural and free movement.

Young kids think nothing of crawling, rolling, moving to and from the ground as part of their interaction with the world, and neither should we. Exploring the limits of our physical freedom has a profound effect on our emotional well being and helps develop a positive and enquiring outlook. That, and the increased mobility, is what helps keep the negative aspects of ageing at bay!

So how should we approach floor work? The first thing is to determine what sort of surface we are working on. If possible, at first I advise you work on mats or, at least, a soft carpet. The floor is very good at pointing out where any tension is in the body and this may be a little uncomfortable to start. As your body relaxes, you can move to a harder surface. In regular class we usually work on a wooden floor, or for the more experienced, outside on all types of surface.

Some exercises can be done on the spot but as you start developing your floor work you will need a little more space. That may mean shifting some furniture around, or, if you have the room, you may be able to set up a full time training area in your home. Another option is to work outside on the lawn- that gets the neighbours talking!

I'd recommend before doing anything, simply lay on the ground and work through any of the breathing exercises from before. Then slowly begin stretching, twisting the arms and legs and moving around a little. Once you have acclimatised yourself you can begin to work.

Approach floor work as all the other exercises. Take your time, monitor the Four Pillars, work within your CRM and repetition limits. As you grow more confident, string some of the exercises and movements together and become more creative in your work. At a further level you can add in obstacles or items to work under, around or through with also.

Before we do anything, let's look at how we can get to the ground easily and safely. There are different ways of doing this, some more challenging than others, but we will start with something nice and gentle! From there we will work into the basic movement methods.

GROUND MOVEMENT

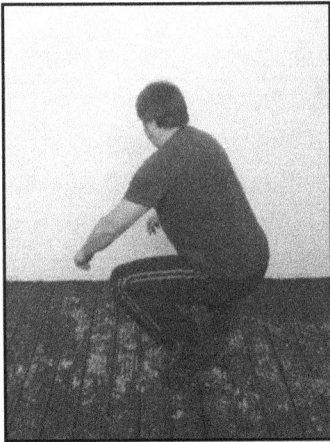

From standing, sink down
into a Cossack squat.

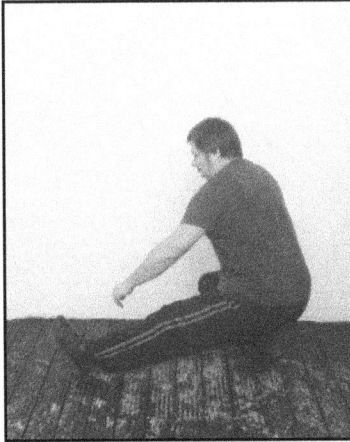

Shift the weight into one leg
and push the other leg out,
foot resting on the heel.
Lower the butt to the floor.

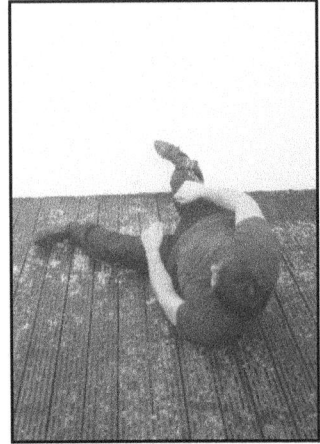

Now allow the body to
softly fall on its side. You
can use the hands but do
not brace the arms!

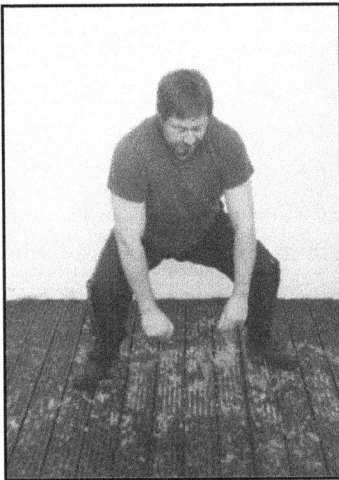

To get down onto your
front, begin from standing
position and again work
down into a Cossack squat.

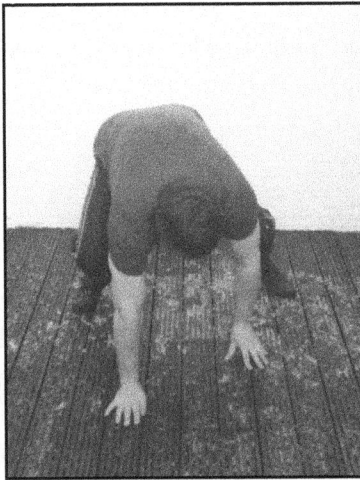

Bring the palms forward
onto the floor and lean
forward, bringing most of
your weight into them.

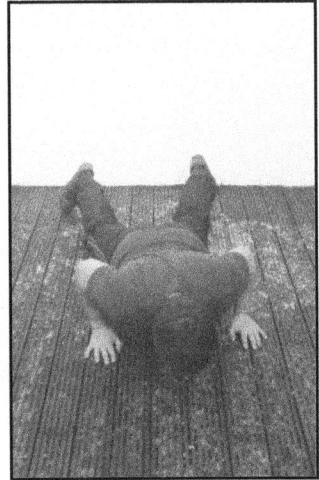

Relax the hips and slide or
"hop" your toes back. You
should now be in low push
up position.

GROUND MOVEMENT

CRAWLING

Lay prone on the floor, on your front, back and side. From each position simply move yourself backwards, forwards and sideways. You can use any/all parts of the body in order to move yourself around. The simplest is as pictured above, on your front use the arms to pull and the legs to push. Use as little tension as possible and remember to keep breathing!

For the next level of challenge, try the same thing but this time you have to keep the body away from the ground. So you can support yourself on hands, elbows, knees and feet as you move forward, sideways and back. Remember not to let the back sag!

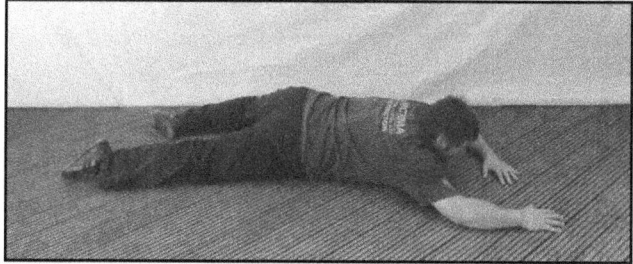

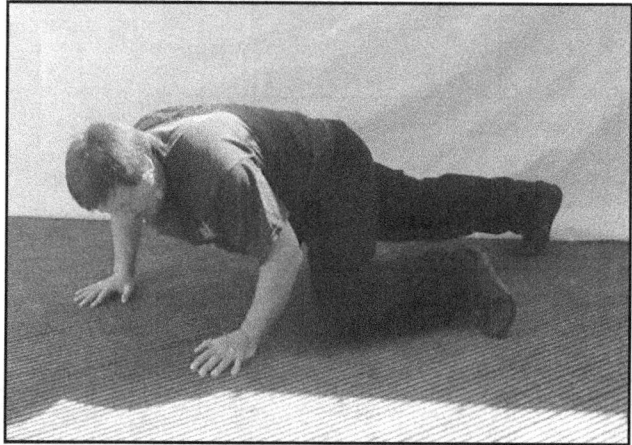

ISOLATED MOVEMENT

You can also try isolated ground movement. Lay flat on your back and move just by rotating the shoulders. Once you get the idea, work different parts of the body - use only the legs, or the arms, for example.

After working on your back, flip over and try the same movements on your front. Think back to the Joint Rotation exercises and you will soon get the idea!

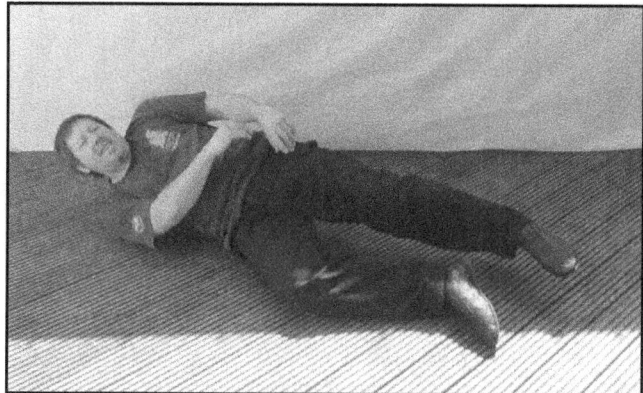

GROUND MOVEMENT

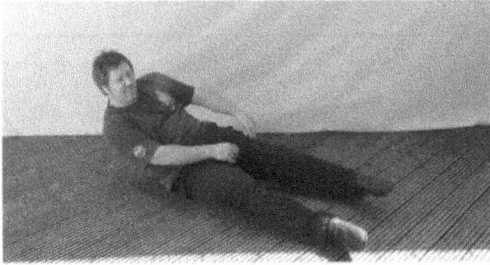

BODY WALKING

Try "walking" using different parts of the body. This can take a little work but is great both for joint rotation and core strength. Try to use only the amount of muscle / tension that you need too. Keep everything else relaxed.

From a sitting position, lift your feet off the ground and walk on your butt. Rotate your hips to move!

Get into a leg raise position and hold it for a couple of seconds. Then start to rotate the shoulders and walk backwards and forwards on them.

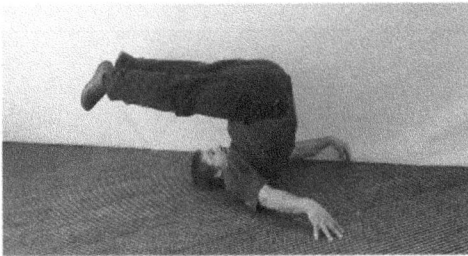

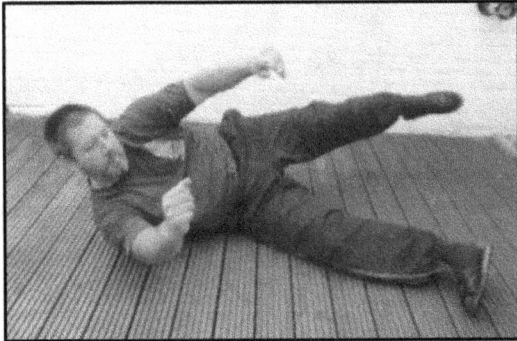

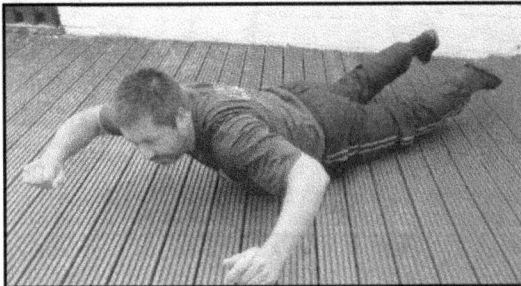

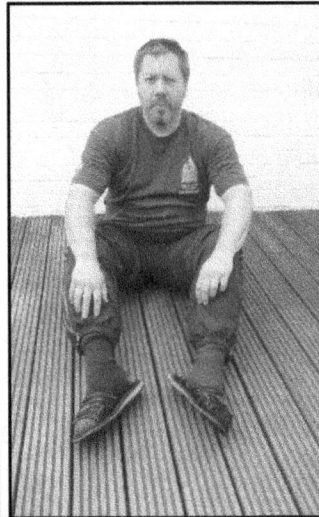

SIT TO FRONT

Sit upright, inhale. As you exhale, pivot by swinging your legs back and reaching your arms forward. Arch the back in order to keep the face from the floor. From the "parachute" position, inhale, then exhale as you lift the arms and pivot again, swinging the legs to the front in order to return to the start position.

GROUND MOVEMENT

CRAB WALK

From the seated position, lean back and place your palms on the floor. Raise your butt and begin walking around in all directions. Keep the breathing working and the body as relaxed as possible.

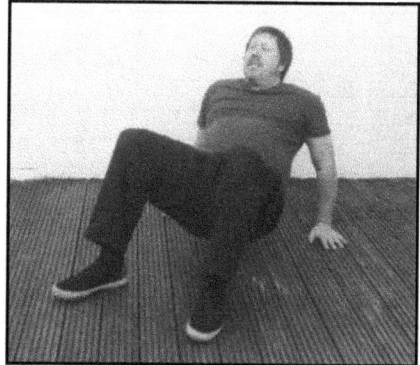

BEAR WALK

From the Crab Walk, turn over onto your hands and toes. Once again, move around in all directions. You can experiment with changing the angle of the body and by placing the hands or feet in different positions.

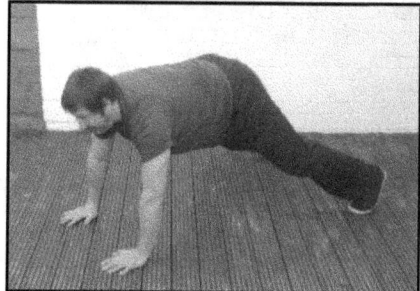

BREAK DANCE

Stay on the hands and toes. Now bring your right foot under and through and stretch the left hand out towards it. Bring hand and foot back to start position and repeat on the other side.

Once you can do that movement smoothly, see if you can continue it. So, this time you continue turning the body and swing the right hand over to contact the floor. In other words, you go from Bear Walk to Crab Walk and back again.

You can then combine all three exercises, move around a little in Bear Walk, do a few Break Dance, then flip over into Crab Walk and move around again.

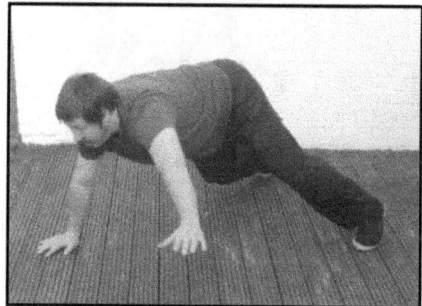

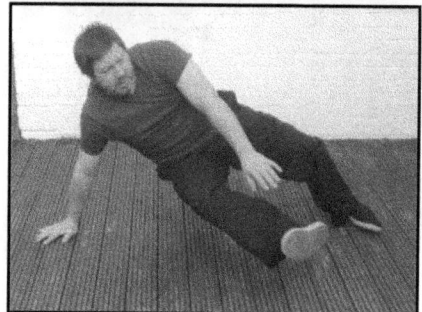

GROUND MOVEMENT

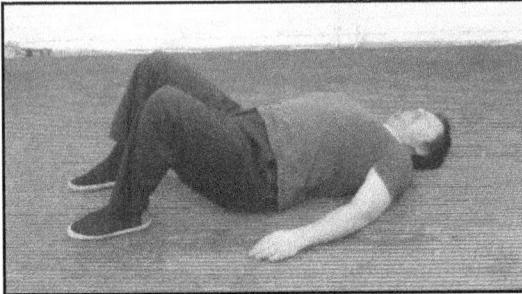

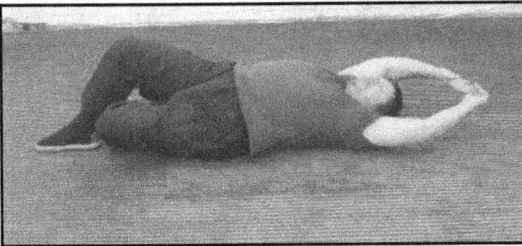

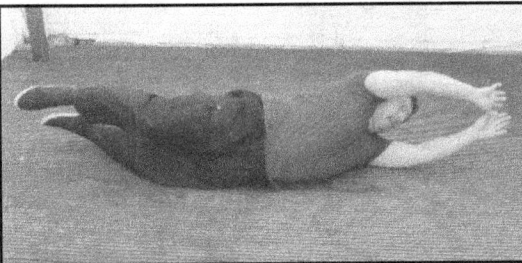

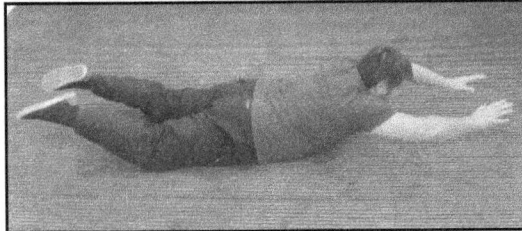

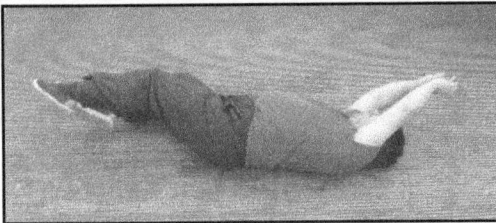

SIDE ROLL

Let's now look at some methods of rolling. The Side Roll is the best one to start with, it is also a very good exercise for stretching the back.

All rolling should be done slowly and smoothly on a suitable surface. The most important thing is to keep the hard, bony areas of the body away from the ground and to always engage with the ground gradually. Keep the muscles relaxed and breathe.

Start by laying on your back with the knees raised. Thread the left foot under and through the right knee.

Use the movement of the foot to turn the body. Stretch the hands out and lift the feet from the floor. Arch the back a little - think of making the body a cylinder.

Continue the movement, allowing the body to roll onto its front, then round onto the back again. If you push the foot out hard enough you will generate enough momentum to roll smoothly. Once you reach the back, repeat on the other side. As far as breathing goes, exhale on the roll.

GROUND MOVEMENT

PUSH UP ROLL

Start in push up position. Rotate your left palm upwards, so bending the elbow and lowering the shoulder to the floor.

Engage the ground smoothly with the shoulder, followed by the whole side of the body.

Go into a sideways roll and turn until you are face down again.

From here rotate the right palm to bring yourself up into the push-up position once more. Try and work the up and down movement completely from the arm rotation and not the shoulder muscles.

Repeat in each direction, working back and forth.

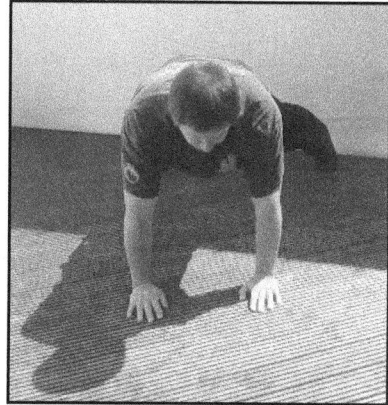

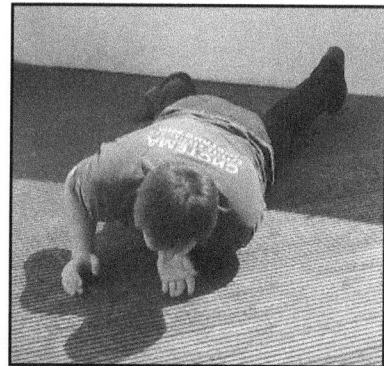

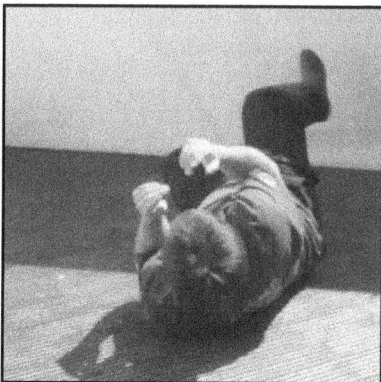

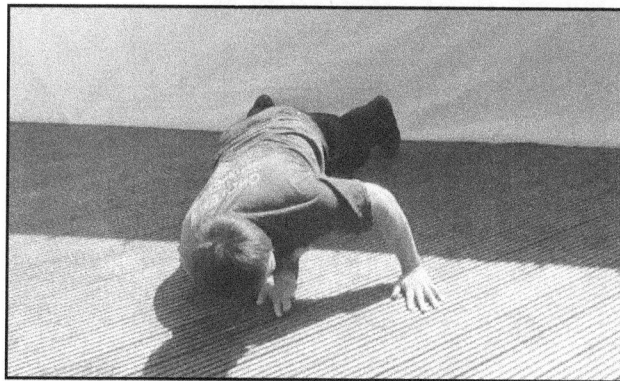

GROUND MOVEMENT

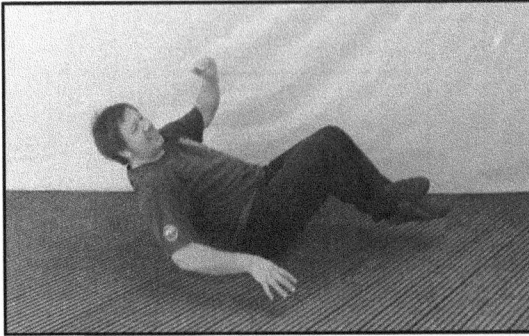

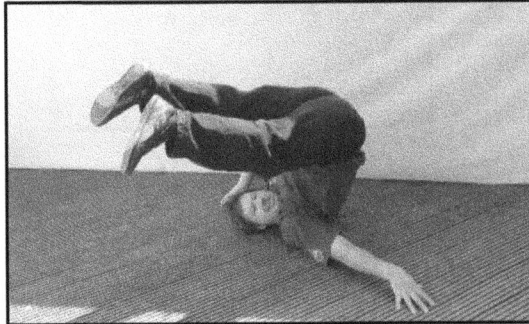

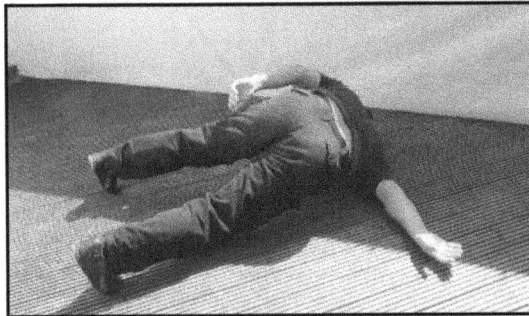

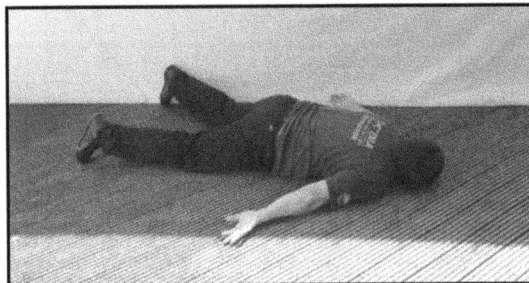

BACK ROLL

From a sitting position, slowly fall backward onto the side of the body. Think back to our Circle and Up exercise, as the start of the roll is the same. One hand can slide out to the side, in order to bring the side of the body gently to the floor.

As you fall back, bring the legs over the head, as though you are doing a leg raise. Try this a few times. Then, to perform the complete roll, instead of bringing the feet over the head, take them over the shoulder. The head should be tucked in a little in order to prevent it from contacting the floor.

As the feet get to about 90 degrees, kick out a bit and/or extend your abdomen. This should give you the momentum to roll over the shoulder. The legs continue out and back until the toes touch the floor. The arms can go out to the side.

You should end up face down. Exhale on the roll. Go slow at first as it can take a little while to do a roll properly. Try and make sure you go over the shoulder and not too much out to the side. Also make sure you are not rolling directly down the spine.

GROUND MOVEMENT

FRONT ROLL

Kneel and place your hands on the floor, to form the corners of a square.

Move the hand to bring your shoulder softly to the floor - either sweep the hand across under you, or slide the hand to the outside. Either way, the shoulder should transition to the floor smoothly.

Tuck the head in towards the opposite knee. Remember, we are trying to keep the back of the head from touching the floor.

Push off with the feet to bring them up and over the head. Again, we are rolling over and across the shoulders, not down the spine. Let the legs swing over and tense the core a little in order to slow their descent. Roll back down to prone position on the side of the body.

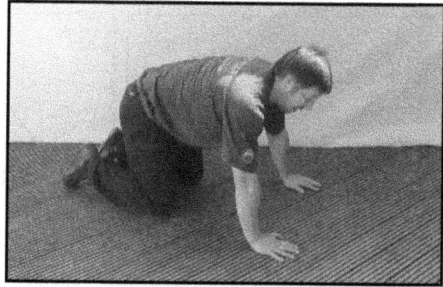

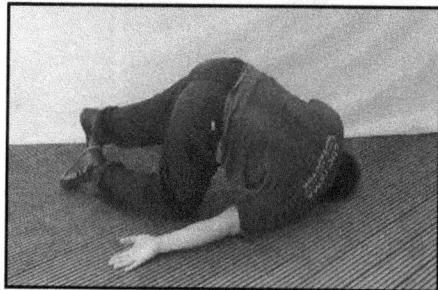

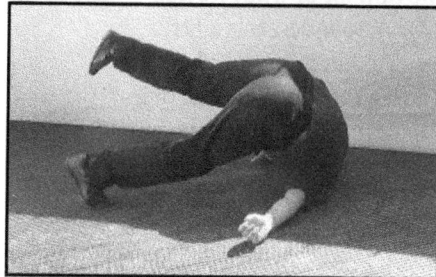

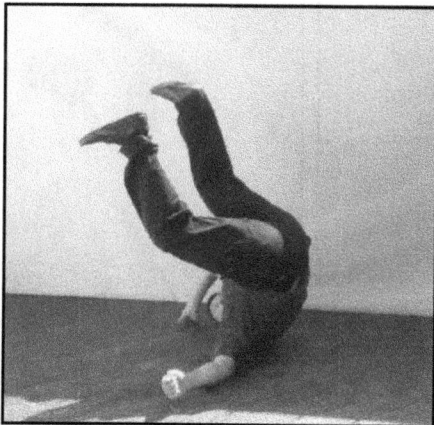

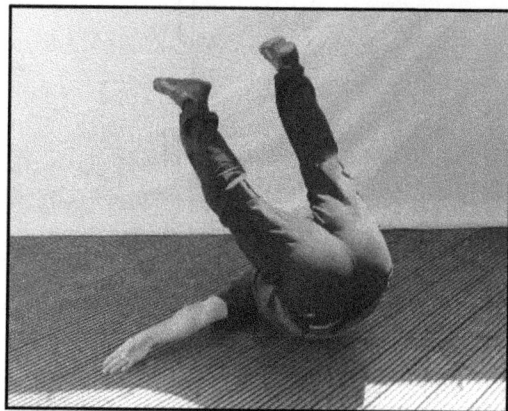

GROUND MOVEMENT

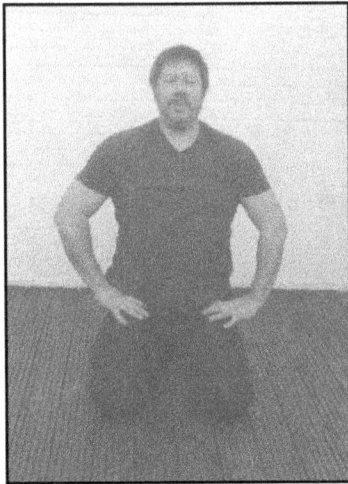

Our last ground exercise is the Knee Walk, a foundation movement of what we call Low Acrobatics. It is a little involved, but is a great drill for opening the hips and working the core. Start by kneeling.

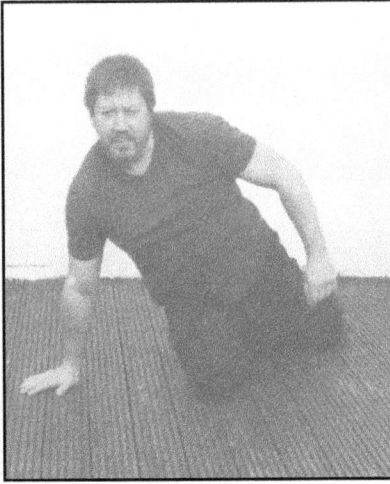

Support yourself with the right hand and shift your weight to the right leg. Slide the left leg back.

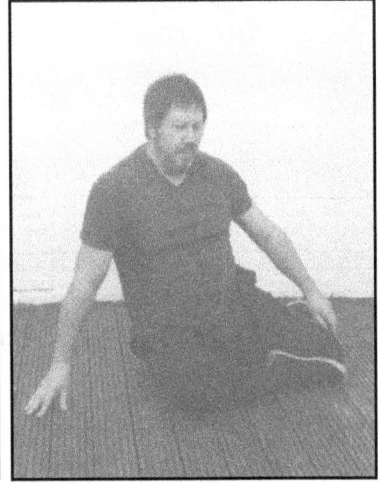

Sit down to the right. Keep the left leg bent behind and position the sole of the right foot to on top of the left knee. This is a great resting position. Use hands for support if required.

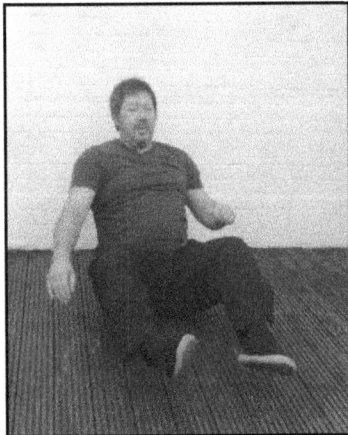

Rock the weight back and, by turning the hips, switch the leg position.

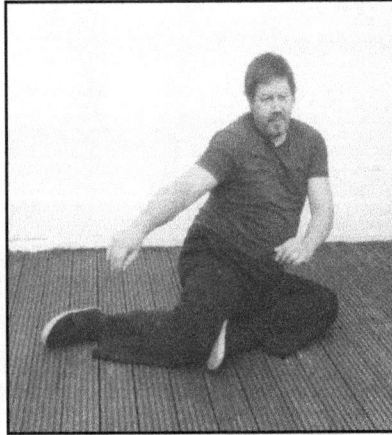

So you then have the left sole on top of the right knee. Again, use the hands if needed.

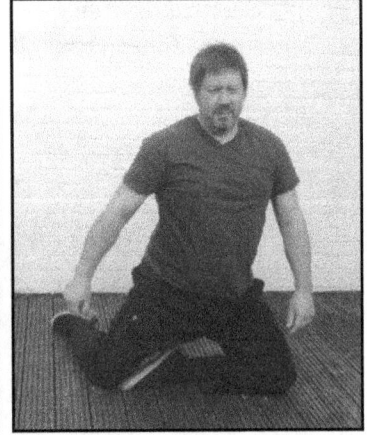

Now open the chest out and pull the body up, lifting so you are sitting on the shins.

GROUND MOVEMENT

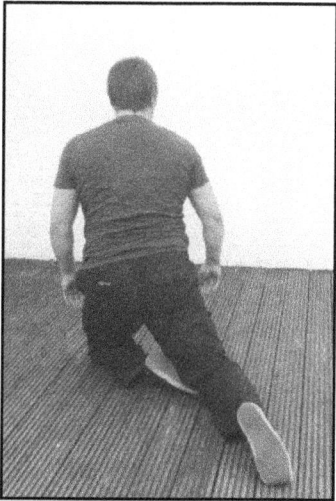

Here's the rear view, left leg in front. Raise up, keep the body straight.

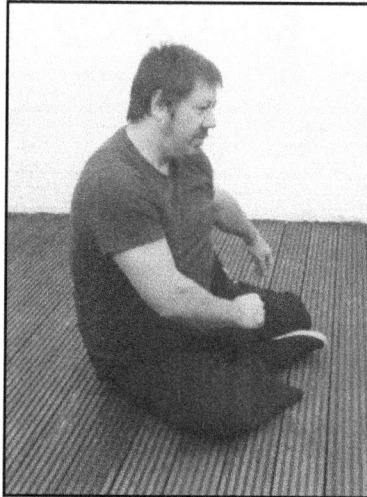

Keeping upright, swivel the legs so that they switch position. The left foot goes out to the side, the right foot slides in.

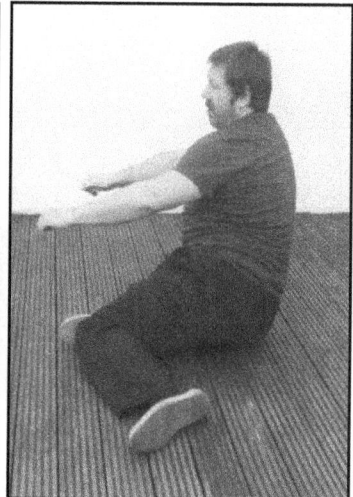

Sit the weight back down and tuck the sole of the right foot onto the left knee.

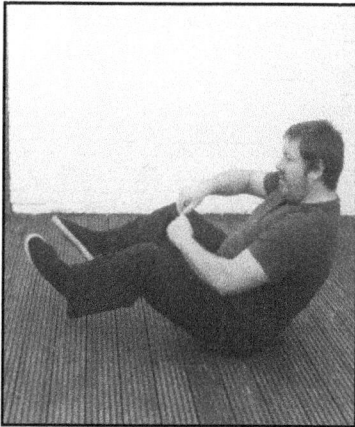

Rock back and switch leg position again.

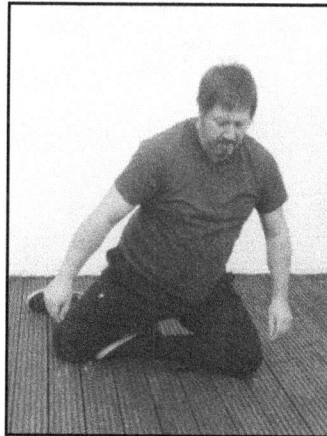

Raise up onto the shins

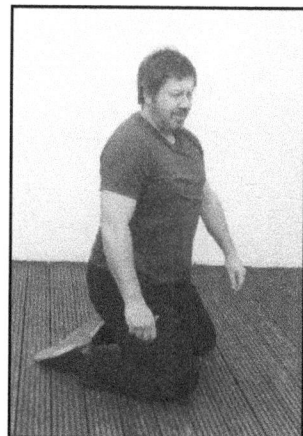

You can finish by returning to start position, or keep cycling through to move across the floor, you can also change direction.

CHAPTER EIGHT

RESISTANCE

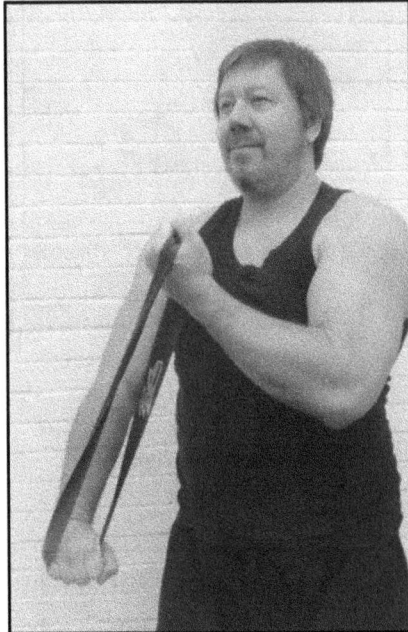

RESISTANCE

Resistance training is as old as the hills. Or at least as old as the rocks and logs on the hills that some early human tried to lift above their head! Resistance training simply involves working against some kind of force in a movement. Bodyweight exercises are just that, we are working purely against the bodyweight (and gravity). Adding an external source of resistance brings many benefits. It builds muscle mass and increases bone density and helps us understand body mechanics.

In days of old people used all kinds of things for resistance training. Some people still use things like large logs , rocks and the like. People also use weapons, or more specialised equipment such as kettle bells, sledge hammers and various forms of weights, such as barbells.

In modern times, gym-based weight training has become the most common form of resistance training. Broadly speaking,there are two types- fixed and free. Fixed weights are the machines you see in the gym. You take up position and move the weight in a fixed pattern. The equipment is designed in such a way that it will not move out of position, giving a lot of stability in the movement.

This kind of work is primarily used to sculpt muscle. It allows for very specific areas of the body to be worked on, so easily allows you to build routines. On the downside, you of course, need access to the equipment! If you don't like the gym environment, you need a lot of space at home to use it all. Another negative, from our movement based perspective, is that the exercise is so isolated. It can introduce a lot of tension into areas of the body and so compromise mobility.

Free weights are exactly how they sound. Something you pick up that is not attached to anything, like a set of dumbbells, for example. Free weights do not have the stability, so on the downside you have to be more careful using them. Though that may be a positive as this forces you to be more aware of your posture!

That lack of stability also works in our favour in terms of strength development. We work the small stabiliser muscles around the joints - and that is where true strength lies, not in the big "for show"muscles! We will cover the use of various type of weight in a future book. To start our resistance training, we will look at stretch bands.

STRETCH BANDS

Stretch bands are an ideal way to start resistance training. They are cheap, easily available and very portable!. We will be working with a short band but longer bands work just as well. The bands come in different thickness, each giving a different level of resistance. Start out with what is comfortable and work your way up. As always, monitor the Four Pillars throughout!

UPPER BODY

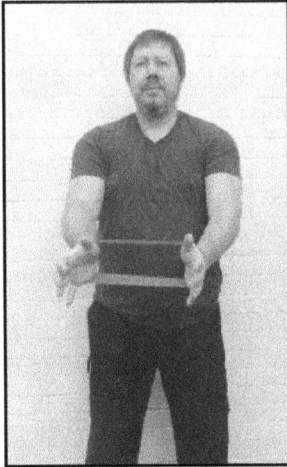

Place the band over the wrists and move them apart until there is just a little tension. Exhale.

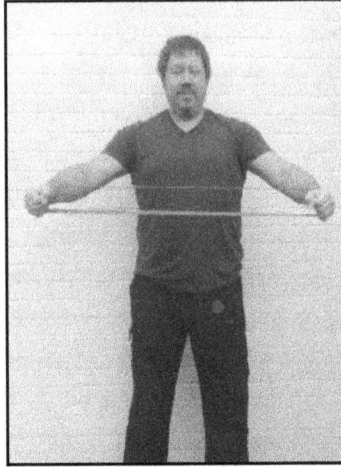

Inhale and pull the hands apart. Allow the chest to expand and tense the core slightly. Exhale and return to start position.

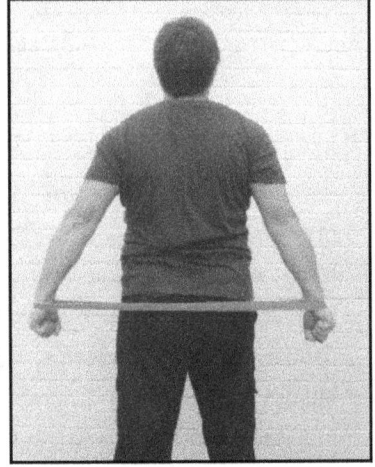

Repeat the same exercise but with the hands behind you.

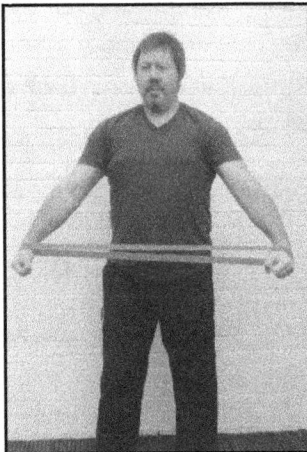

Remember the selective tension exercise from the Stick Exercises? We can do exactly the same movement with the band.

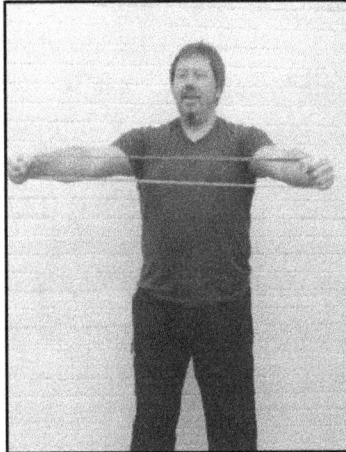

Bring the hands out and maintain the tension as you slowly lift.

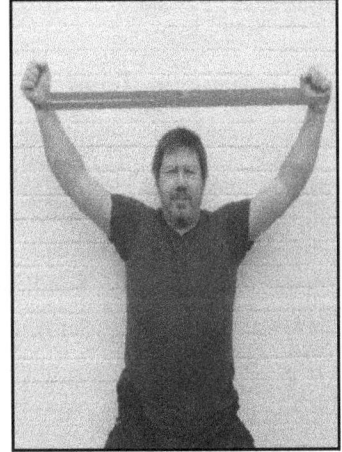

Raise the hands above the head. Relax, then reapply tension and lower to start point. Burst breath throughout.

UPPER BODY

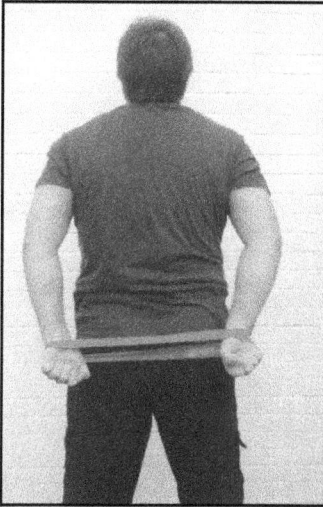

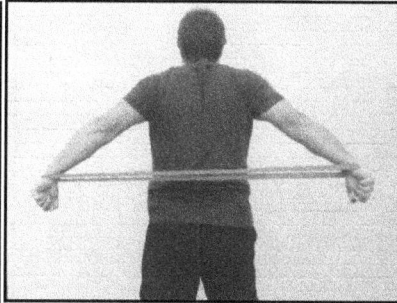

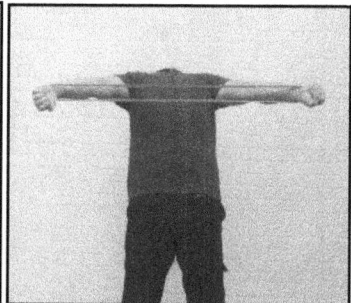

Repeat the same procedure to the rear. Lean the head forward a little if necessary to get a bit more lift. Experiment also with holding the fully stretched band in various positions for a short time.

Hold the band as shown, with one palm down, one up. Inhale. Exhale as you pull the top hand up. Inhale and return to the start point. Repeat as required then switch the hands over.

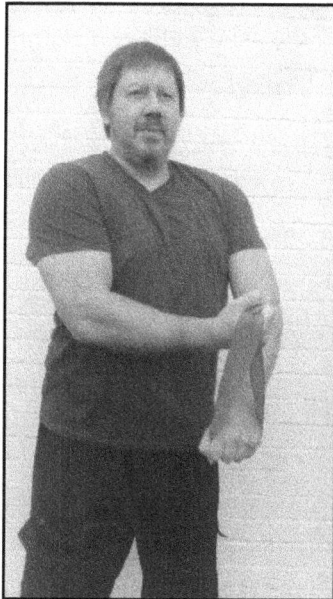

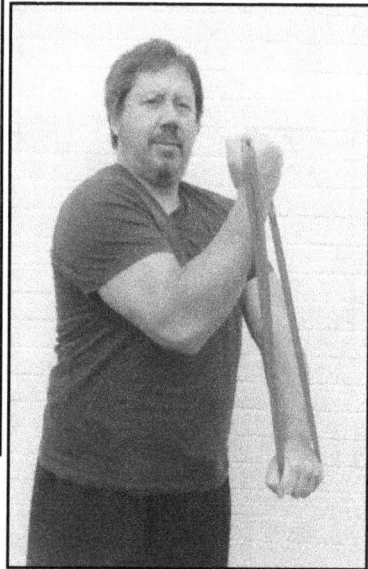

UPPER BODY

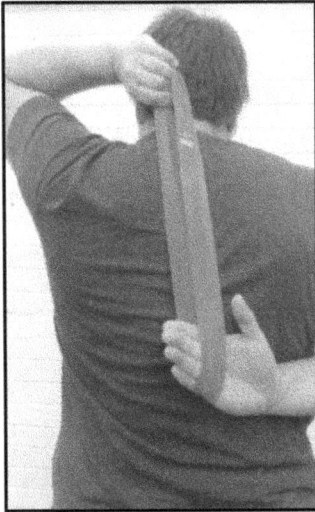

Lift one hand behind the head and hang the band down the back. Grab it with the other hand. Inhale.

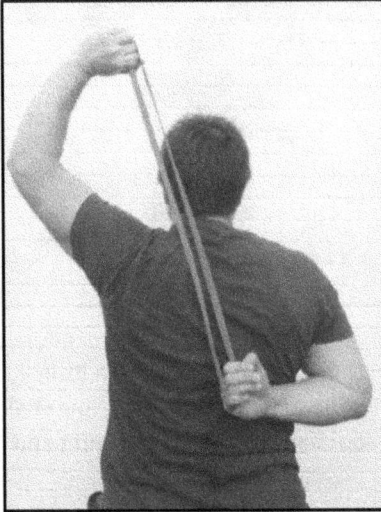

Exhale and pull the top hand, keeping a firm grip on the band with the lower hand.

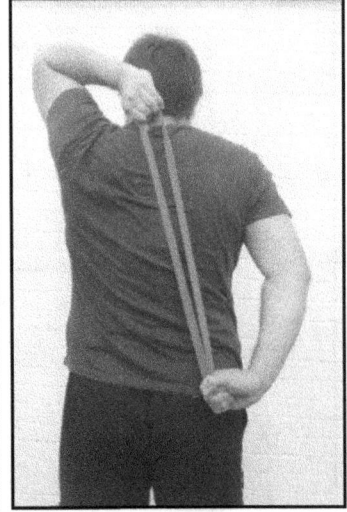

Reverse the exercise by grasping the band in the top hand and pulling down with the lower hand.

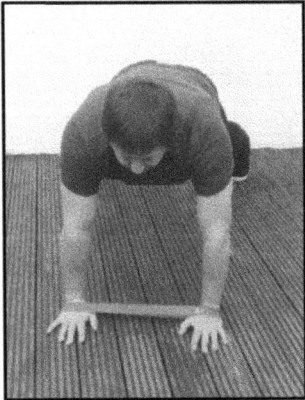

Get into push up position with the band over the wrists.

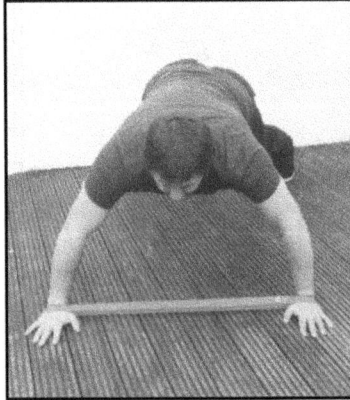

Bring the hands out to the sides and perform a push up. When you come back up, bring the hands in again.

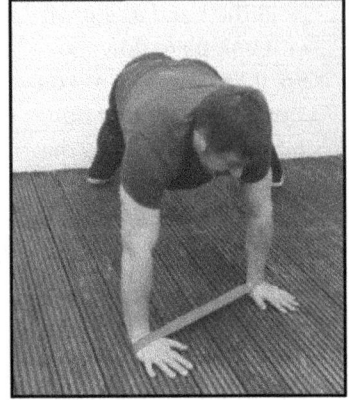

From the same start point, move the hands around into different positions, maintaining tension in the band.

LEGS

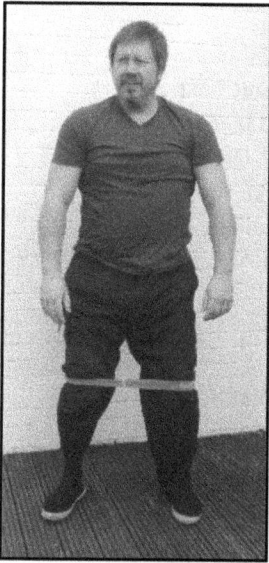

Place the band outside
of the knees.
Remember to remove it
if the phone rings…

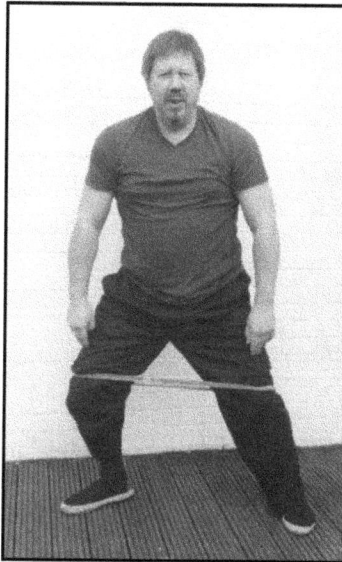

Take one foot out to
the side on the exhale.
Squat down a little into
the movement.

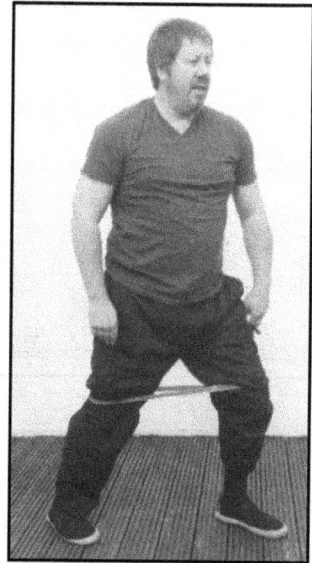

Come back to the start
point and repeat on the
other side.

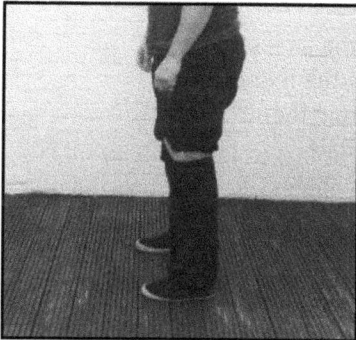

From the same start
point you can also step
backwards and
forwards.

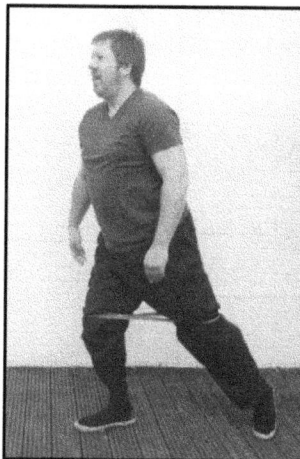

Experiment with
keeping the moving
foot flat or lifted.

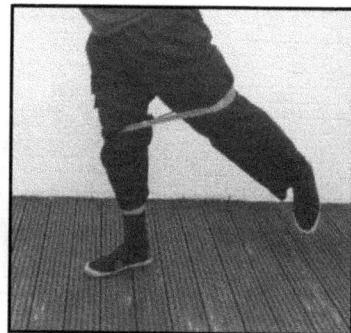

Or try lifting the moving
foot completely off
of the ground.

LEGS

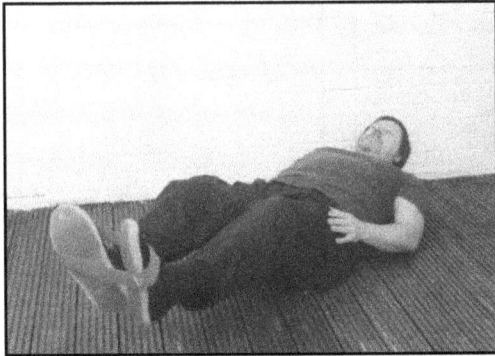

Next, lay on your back with the band placed over your feet. Lift the feet just off of the ground and inhale.

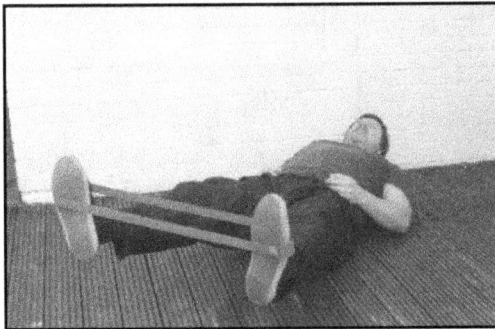

Exhale and pull the feet apart as wide as you can. Keep the shoulders on the floor. Inhale and return to start.

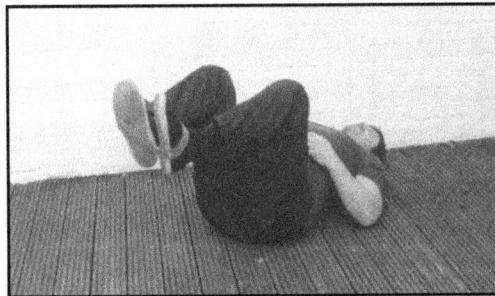

Now pull the knees up and bring the feet in close together. Inhale.

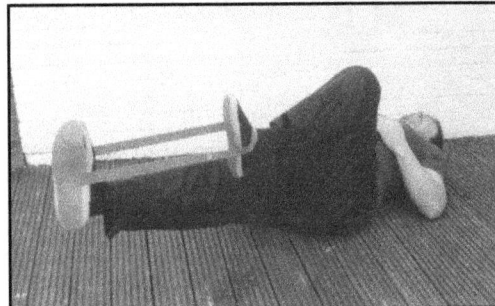

Push one foot away as you exhale. Inhale and bring it back to start.

LEGS

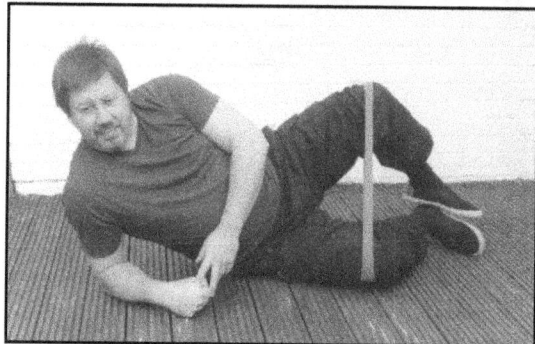

Roll over onto your side and bring the band up around the ankles. Inhale.

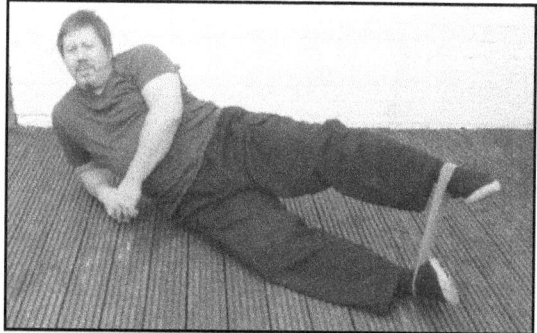

Exhale and lift the top foot as high as you can. Inhale and return to start position.

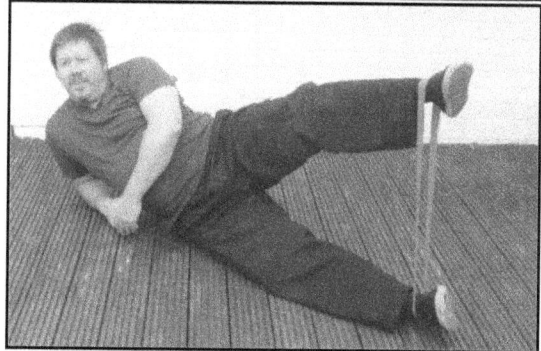

Stay on your side and bring the band up around the knees. Inhale.

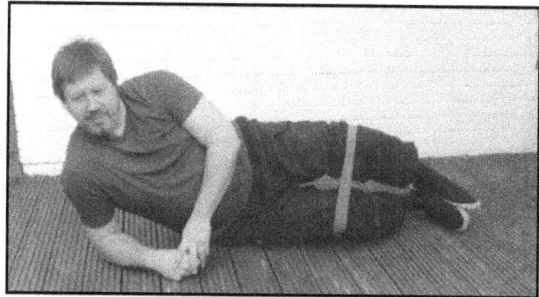

Exhale and rotate the top knee outwards. Alternatively, you can left the whole leg. Inhale and return to start.

CHAPTER NINE

PROGRESSION

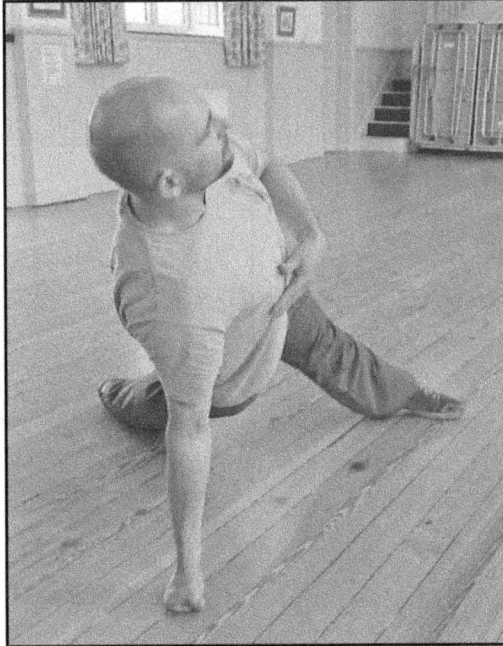

PROGRESSION

We have now covered the basic exercises and I'm sure there is enough there to keep you busy for a while! However, I am a firm believer in keeping exercise as interesting as possible. Exercise can become a dull routine or chore if we are not careful, plus we also need to give the body fresh challenges if we are to keep growing.

Now "challenges" in some exercise regimes simply mean going faster, doing more reps, lifting heavier weights, all with the attendant risk of injury. Instead, we can look at small ways to change our basic exercises in order to make our body work in a slightly different way to perform them. New movement means forming new neural pathways, which in turn helps with keeping our mind and body fresh and active.

We can work these variations in two different ways. First of all, I will show some different ways to do the basic exercises, to give you a few examples. Then I will describe the Formula that was previously mentioned. With this key knowledge under your belt you will easily be able to make up your own variations. In effect, the Formula gives a method of providing almost countless variants on the original movements.

Combining exercises into *movement chains* is another important aspect of training too. The usual approach is to, say, do some squats, then stop for a minute, then do some push ups and so on. Instead, once you have the basic movements down, I want you to think about how you transition from one exercise to the next. If you have done some sit ups, then perform a side roll to get into push up position. Or go direct from your last squat into a plank position. This way you will also begin to develop *flow* in your work.

FLOW

Flow is a very interesting concept and one that is absent from most fitness routines, though of course it is strongly present in martial arts and dance disciplines. On a simple level, we can think of flow as smooth movement; not jerky, minimal tension, gliding, like a cat. That is certainly one level, but the concept of flow goes rather deeper. Here's how a friend of mine, Bruno Caverna of *Formless Arts* describes it:

"Everything is whole and working together, there is only the moment, the moment is only for itself. Nothing exists outside what you are doing here and now, you just do what needs to be done, be, exist. You do think and feel on some level, but with only your body and unconscious mind (a lot faster and smoother). This is where the real learning occurs."

Flow, then, is as much as state of mind as a physical thing. We have all experienced it at some time, that feeling of being in the zone,

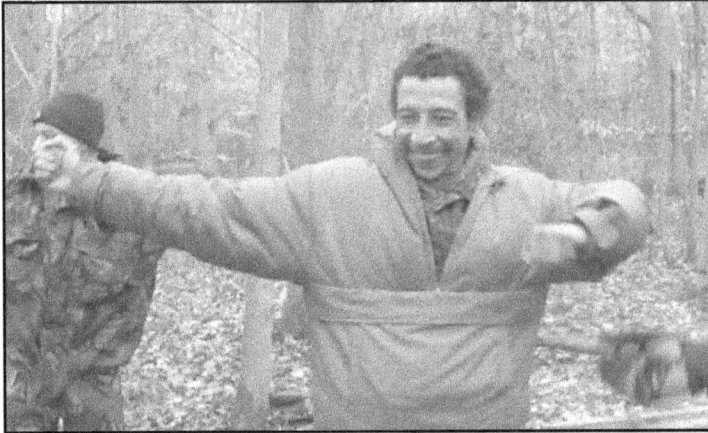

where everything just clicks, there is no conscious effort involved. I've experienced it playing music, in martial arts training and in a few dangerous situations. My Russian teachers refer to this state as *professional mindset*, the actions a person such as a paramedic, soldier, nurse, etc takes in extreme situations. They don't panic, they just do what needs to be done.

The interesting thing for me is I have found that teaching people flowing movement significantly helps them to gain that flowing mindset. There is a deeper level of brain-body engagement when your exercise is focused, when your movement is mindful, that you just don't get by blasting out reps to loud music.

How do we develop that mindfulness? The breathing is key. It sounds so simple, yet all the breathing methods described in this book will bring you to a deeper level of mind-body coordination which in turn will help you flow.

So be aware of your breathing throughout and work to move smoothly when exercising, but also when transitioning between exercises. Carry that over into your daily life and you will find your movement becomes efficient, effective and fun!

There is a Psychology Professor who, after certain experiences in World War Two, devoted much time to studying the Flow State. His name is Mihaly Csikszentmihalyi. After carrying out extensive research he formulated what he calls the *Eight Characteristics of Flow*, as follows:

1. Complete concentration on the task
2. Clarity of goals and reward in mind and immediate feedback
3. Transformation of time , speeding up/slowing down of time
4. The experience is intrinsically rewarding
5. Effortlessness and ease
6. There is a balance between challenge and skills
7. Actions and awareness are merged, losing self-conscious rumination
8. There is a feeling of control over the task

If you are interested in exploring this topic further I recommend the Professor's work. You can Google him to find out more (and don't worry, I don't know how to pronounce his name either!).

Now, let's start with some of the core exercise variations, beginning with push ups.

VARIATIONS

PUSH UP, HANDS AND FEET

Start in the basic push up position. The first variation is simply to adjust the width of the hands. Try bringing the hands close together, try moving them as far apart as you can. Be aware that with the latter movement there can be considerably more strain on the shoulders, so proceed with care.

Another variation is to start wide and with each push-up, move the hands in a little closer. Once the hands meet, move outward again between each push up. Also try working the hands forward, singly or together.

Experiment also with foot position - move the feet wide, raise one foot and so on.

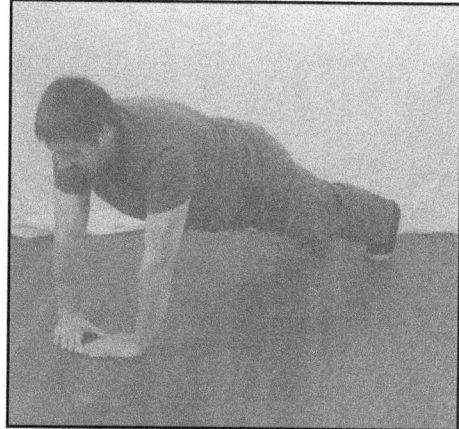

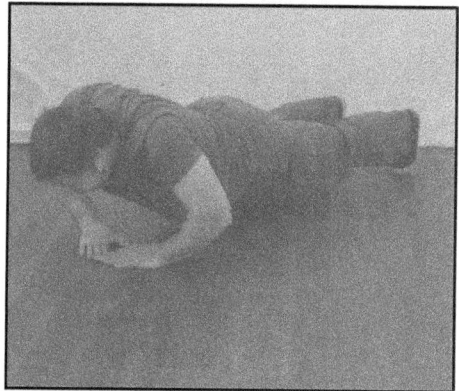

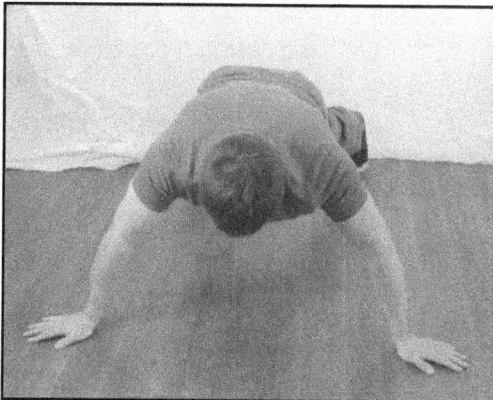

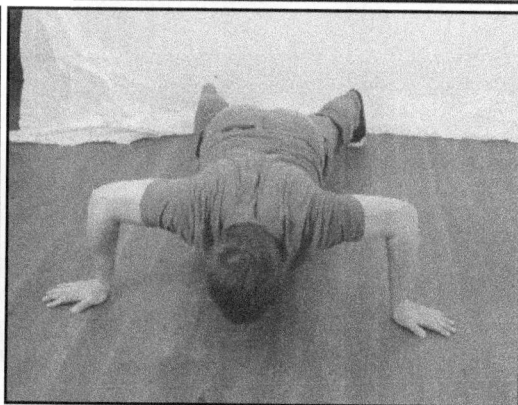

VARIATIONS

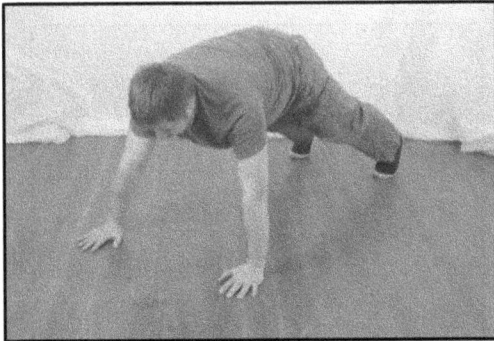

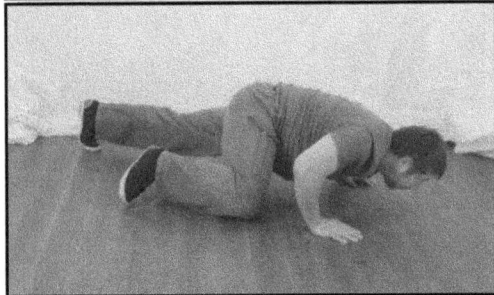

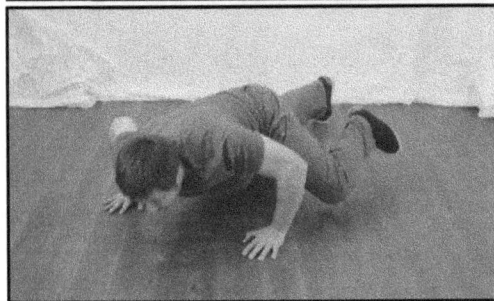

MOUNTAIN CLIMBER PUSH UP

Start in regular pushup position. There are two variations on this exercise. For the first, keeping the back level and the shoulders relaxed, lift one foot and bring the right knee up towards the chest. Immediately bring it back and now take the left knee up towards the chest. It's a little like running on the spot, but with your hands on the ground! You can also try bringing both knees up at the same time.

For the second variation, the toe is again lifted but this time the knee come towards the elbow. As you bring the knee up, you lower the body down as in a regular push up. When the body lifts, the foot goes back to the start position. Repeat on the other side.

ELEVATED PUSH UP

Work a regular push up but with the feet elevated. You can easily use a chair or something similar, as long as it is stable. Once used to the exercises,you can experiment with different hand positions as before.

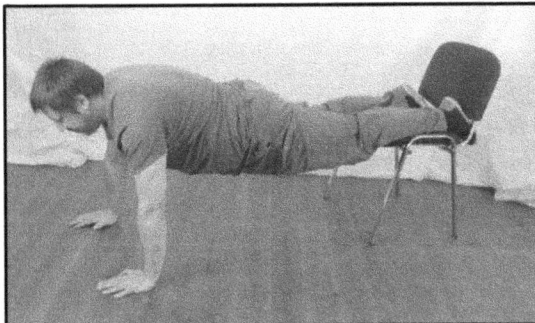

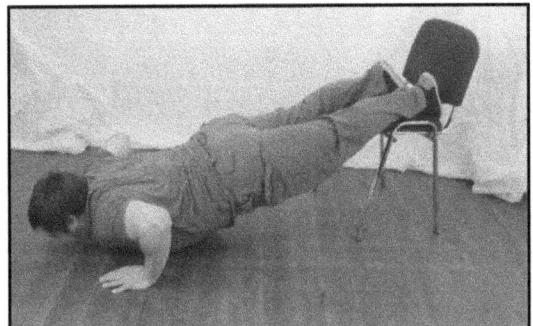

VARIATIONS

DIVE BOMBER PUSH UP

Start in regular pushup position. Make sure your hands are directly under your shoulders. Keep your back level and relax your shoulders.

Separate your feet to at least shoulder-width apart, you can have your feet out much wider than your shoulders if that is more comfortable for you.

Lift your hips up, while keeping your arms and legs as straight as you can. As you do this, contract your abs and push through the area between the back of the shoulders). Your body should create an inverted "V" This is the start position, which you will return to do multiple repetitions of this exercise. You should be standing on your toes or the balls of your feet. Lengthen your hamstrings by pulling down through your heels towards the ground.

Lower your body. Imagine a dot between your hands. As you lower towards the ground, aim to place your nose on that dot. Push the elbows out to either side a little as you lower.

Flatten your body to the ground and slide it forward. The torso should be parallel to the ground but not touching it. This is the halfway point of the movement. From here, circle up, return to the start position and repeat.

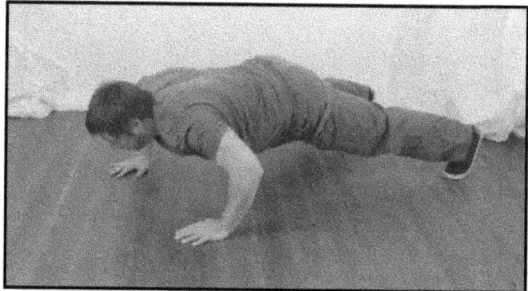

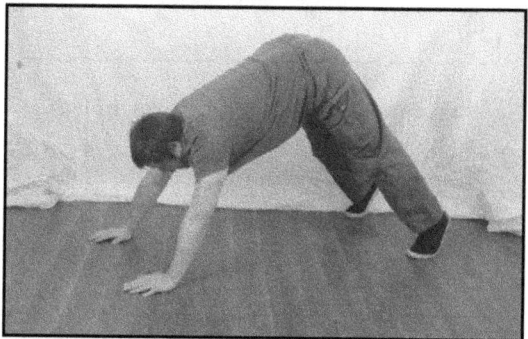

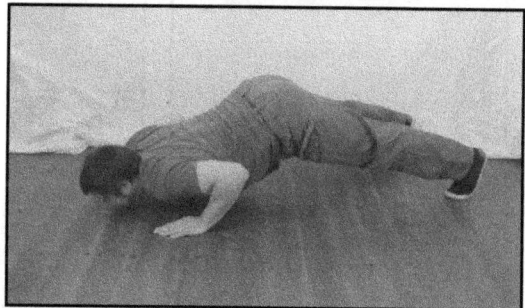

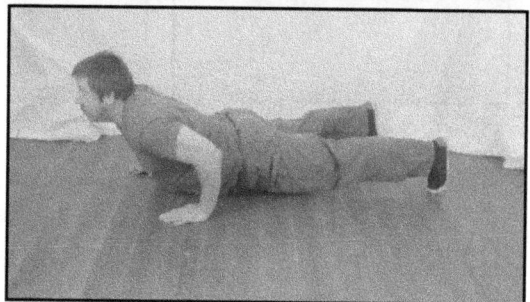

VARIATIONS

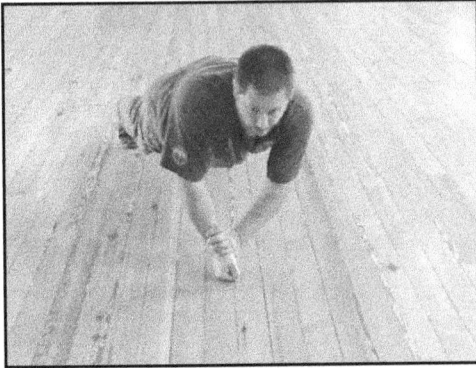

If you are feeling strong, you might like
to try one-arm push ups.
Clasp your wrist with the opposite hand.

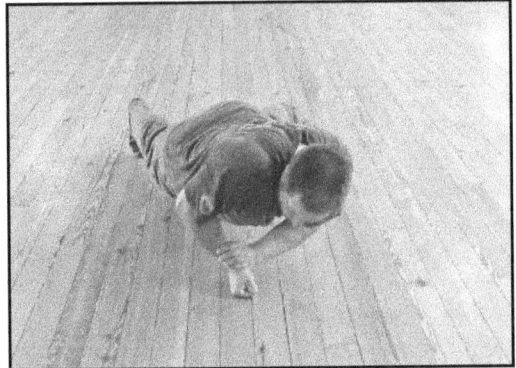

Lower down slowly as you inhale.
Then exhale and push back up.

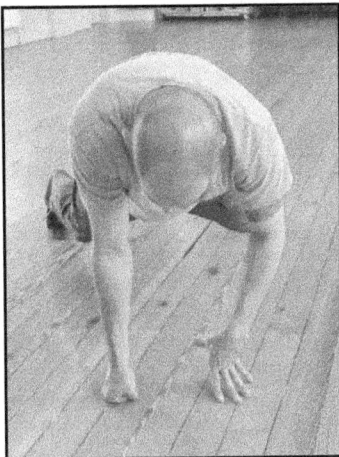

An alternative version is to
start by doing a normal push
up.

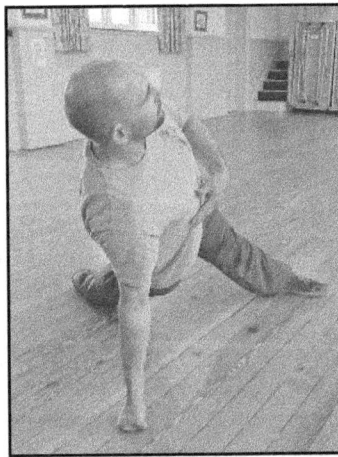

When you come back up, turn
to one side a little. You can
have the feet a little wider.

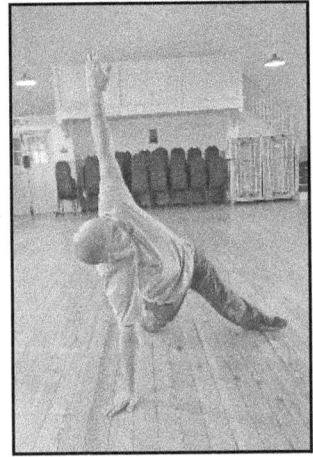

Reach up as high as you can
with the arm, then turn the
body back, bring the hand
down and do another push
up.

VARIATIONS

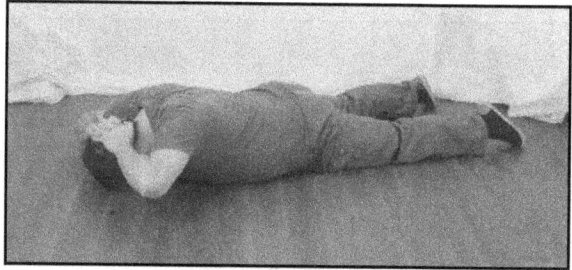

REVERSE SIT UP

Lay on your front and place your hands behind your head. Inhale, then exhale.

As you inhale again, lift the head up, raising the upper body from the floor as high as you can.

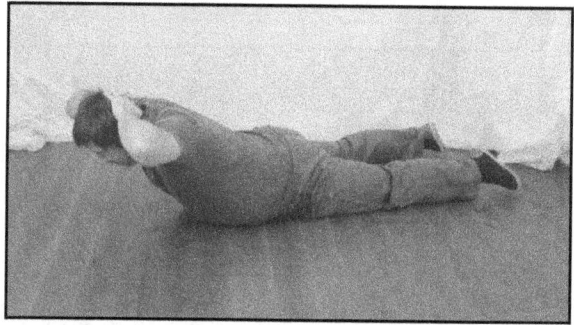

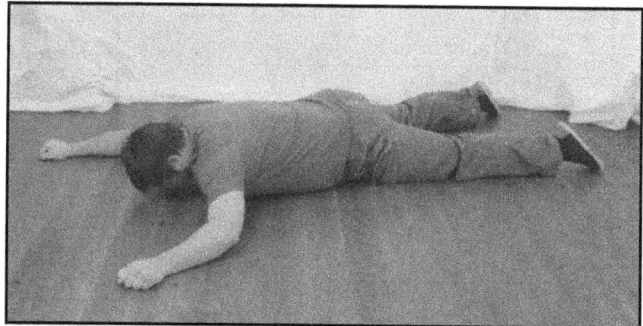

PARACHUTES

Lay on your front and place your hands behind your head. Inhale, then exhale.

As you inhale again, take the head up, raising the upper body and the feet up from the floor as high as you can.

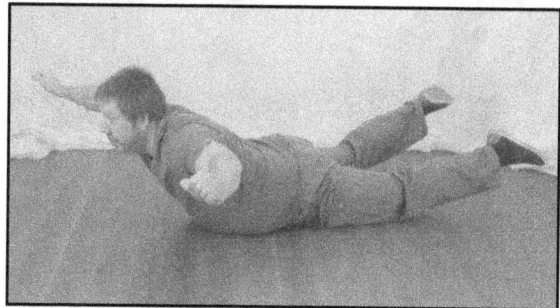

VARIATIONS

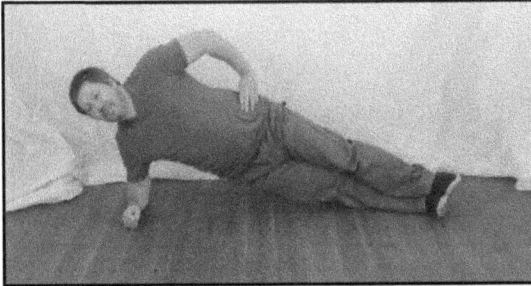

SIDE PLANK

Turn on your side and support the body with forearm and feet. Keep the body straight and hold the position. From here you can also move the hips up and down to work the abs.

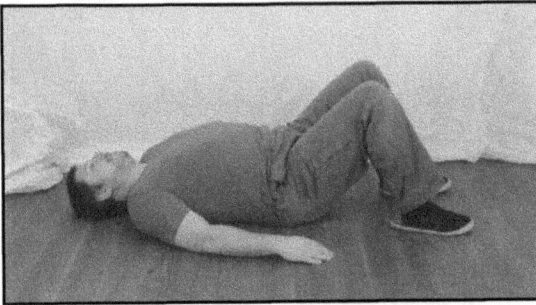

BODY RAISE

Lay on your back, arms at sides and raise your knees. Inhale.

Exhale and raise your hips as high as you can. Keep the feet flat and your shoulders on the floor. Inhale and lower down again.

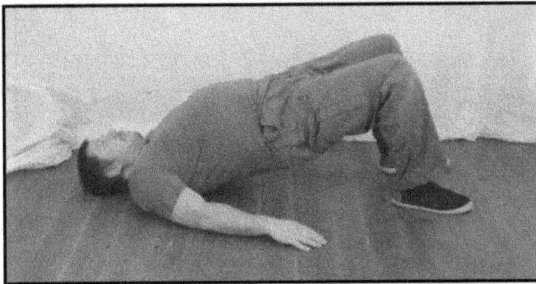

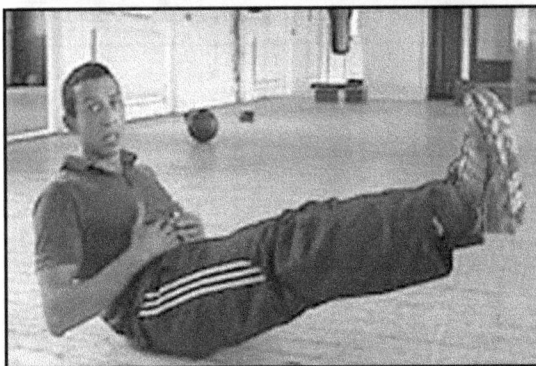

THE V SIT

Lay on your back and inhale. As you exhale, raise both body and feet.

Hold the position for as long as you can while burst breathing. To finish, lower slowly to the floor.

VARIATIONS

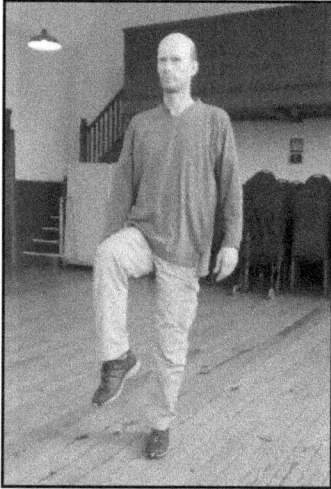

SLOW KICKS

This is a variation on the leg Joint Rotation exercise and is very good for developing stability and balance.

Start by raising one knee as high as you can. Now slowly push the foot out in a kicking movements. Let the supporting leg bend a little at the knee.

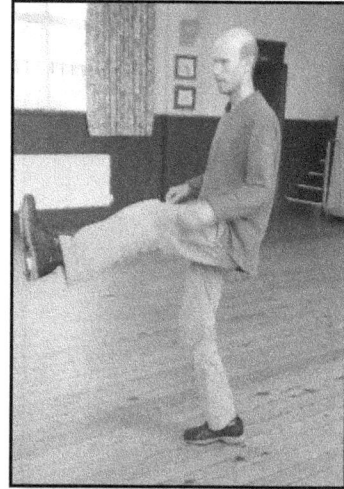

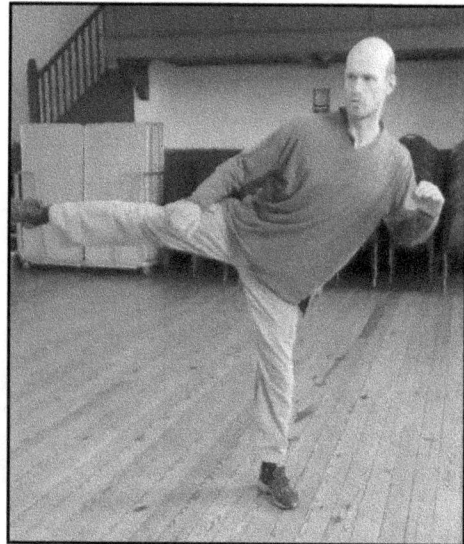

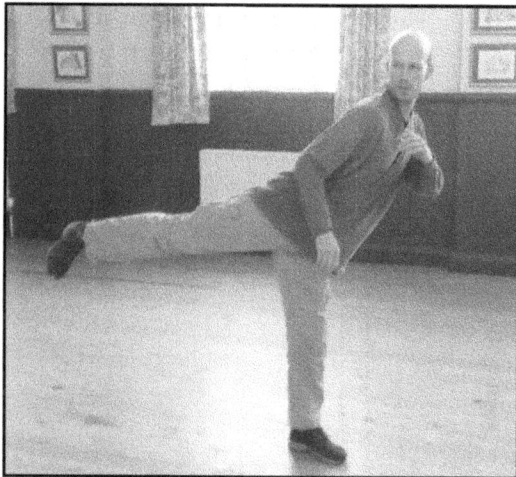

Now make the same kicking move to the rear, without putting the foot down if possible. Continue by kicking out to the sides, left and right. Pivot on the supporting foot if necessary.

You don't have to follow the sequence, you can kick out in any direction. The main thing is to keep your movement slow and smooth and to maintain your balance. Use support or put the foot down if you need to at first.

VARIATIONS

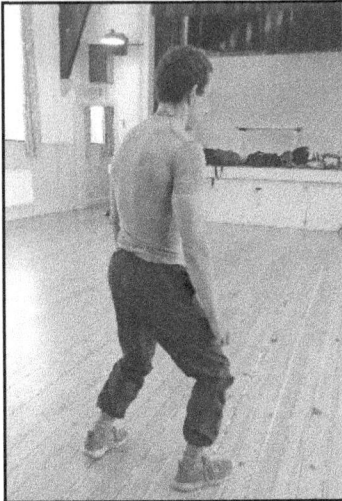

The Cross Legged Squat is another variation. Start in the normal position

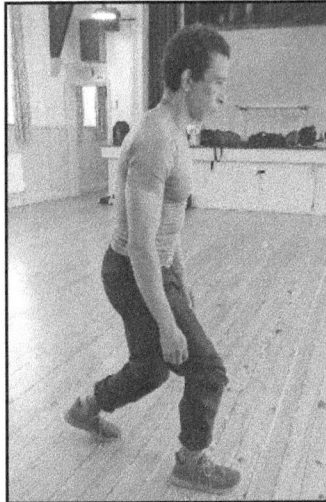

Place your right foot forward and shift your weight into it.

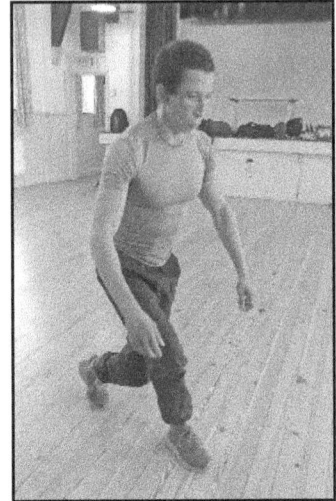

Raise the rear heel as you begin to sink down into the front leg. Check the knee alignment!

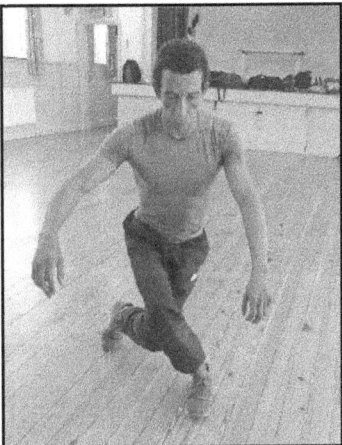

Continue to sink, allowing the rear knee to move forwards. Keep the body upright.

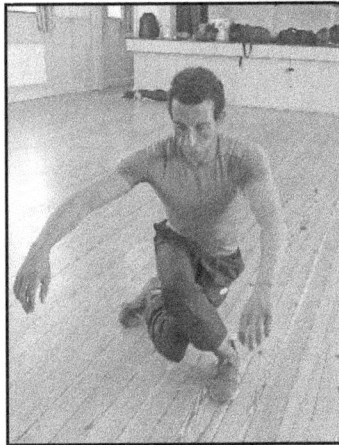

Sit down towards the rear heel. The back toes can slide out a little if required.

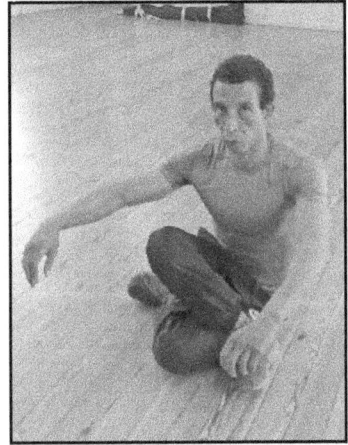

Sit down fully in the cross legged position. Hold for a while then bring the weight forward and slowly stand up.

THE FORMULA

Having looked at some specific variations on our Core Exercises, let's look at our Formula. The Formula is based on the Four Pillars and here's how it works - think of each of the Pillars in turn and how they can be adjusted.

Posture relates to the structure of our body. In simple terms, that means moving our hands and feet into different positions while doing the exercise. So for a squat, start in the normal shoulder width position, then move the feet out a bit wider on each squat. Once you have gone as wide as you can, bring the feet all the way back in on each squat until they are touching.

We can do a similar thing with push ups, moving the hands and feet around in different positions. Try starting with the hands under the shoulders, then move them out a little on each push-up, until they are as far apart as you can manage. Then decrease the distance each time until the hands are touching. You can place them in different positions as you do the push up. Other options are taking a hand or foot of the floor.

For Movement, think of the speed of the exercise and how you can alter it. Try doing the exercise very slowly. For example, perform a squat on a 20 count. One is start position, 20 is full squat. Burst breathe where necessary. The slow exercises are great for building endurance and for highlighting areas of weakness or tension that need further work. When you find a point in the movement that is difficult, try not to rush through it. In fact, it is good to hold in that position for a little while, this way we work on the weakest link in our movement chain!

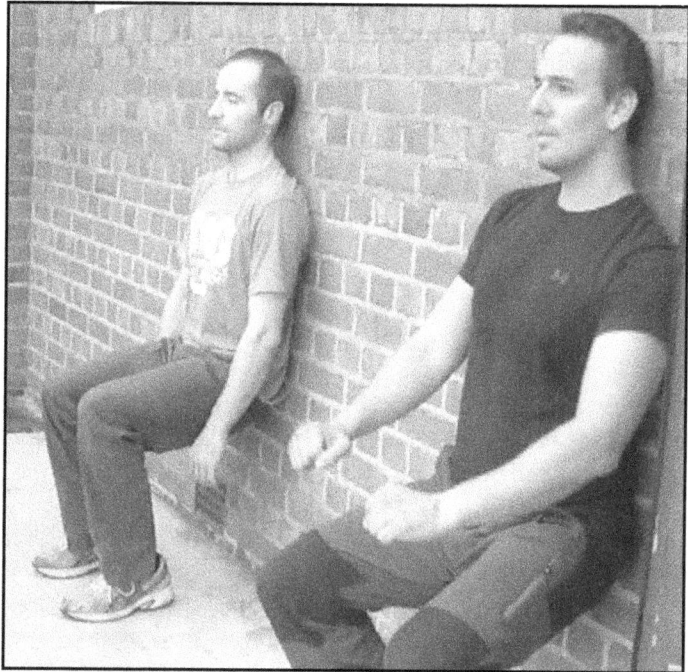

From slow, move to mid-pace and then try as fast as you can. You can either inhale/exhale fast with the movement, or try the Ladder Breathing. For example, do three push ups on an inhale, then three on an exhale. You can also mix fast and slow. Sit up slowly, then drop back down quickly, for example.

Full stop is also a speed variation! We have covered the plank, but you don't have to hold it at the top. Try holding half way down. Ditto for the squat and sit up.

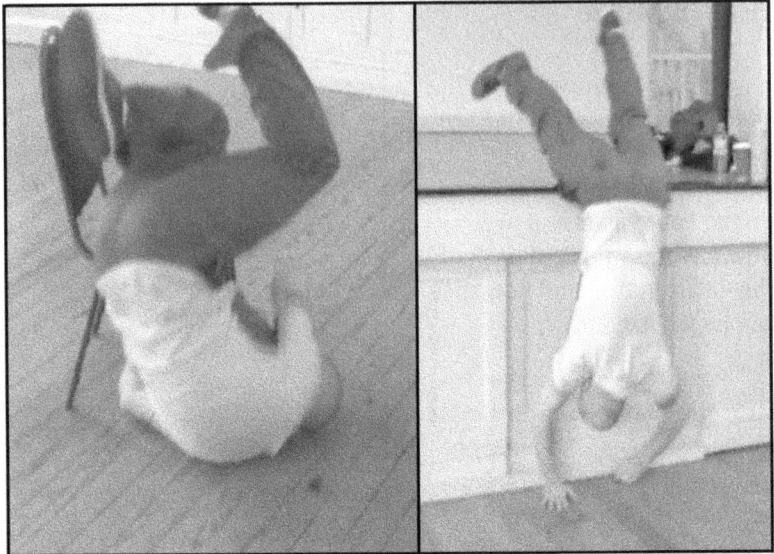

For Relaxation, here are a couple of ideas. Start a squat in a relaxed posture, then as you go down deeper, add in more tension. So at the bottom of the squat, the body is fully tense. As you rise up, relax in time with the movement until you are fully relaxed at the top of the squat. Of course, you can switch this sequence around and use it for the other Core Exercises too. You could also try selective tension during an exercise - just keep one part of the body, say and arm or a leg, tense throughout the movement.

Another option is to try and do the exercises totally relaxed, floppy even. For the push up, sink all the way to the floor and, from that resting position try and raise yourself with absolute minimal use of muscles.

Breathing patterns can be varied in many ways, some we have already discussed. Mix up your inhale /exhale patterns, work the Ladder and Square breathing in with the exercises and generally get a feel for how the breathing can support the movement. Try fast movements with slow breathing and vice versa.

Advanced breathing involves working with extended breath holds, but only after gaining experience in the basic methods. I wouldn't recommend them whilst moving at this stage but you can and should work on extending the static breath hold in your Square Breathing.

So take the Four Pillars as your points of variation and play around with them. I'm sure there are many variations you can find too, particularly once you add a partner into the mix!

EQUIPMENT

It is easy to combine the use of equipment into our Core Exercises. We have already seen how we can use a stick as well as the wall and chairs as support for push ups and squats. Another way to use the wall is to get in press up with the feet close to the wall. Shuffle back and climb the feet up the wall until you are almost in a handstand position. Now work the push ups. You can climb back down or go into a forward roll to come out of the exercise.

You can also add equipment into your Ground Movement work. Use items of furniture as obstacles, crawl around, under and over them. Outdoors, use natural obstacles, trees are also good for climbing. The world is your gym!

The stretch band and stick are easy to incorporate into the Core Exercises. Try performing a squat with the stick placed over the shoulders, for example. This will really help with keeping the spine straight.

Try working the sit up with the stick in the same position. You may well find this very difficult at first, so think about kicking out with the feet in order to lift yourself. A strong exhale on the up move will also help!

From the upright position, you can transition into the Sit to Front exercise. Be sure to keep your shoulders relaxed and keep the face turned to the side as you go forward. Best to work on a soft surface to begin with.

Use any opportunity where you have to carry or lift something heavy to practice your posture and breathing. Remember, knees bend and straight back when lifting!

I mentioned briefly about working with a partner, or even a group of people. We cover this subject in more detail in our *Human Gym* book. In short, look at what you have around you and be creative with how you can incorporate it into your exercise. See how many of your regular actions actually have an exercise component to them and you will soon begin to blur the lines between exercise and activity.

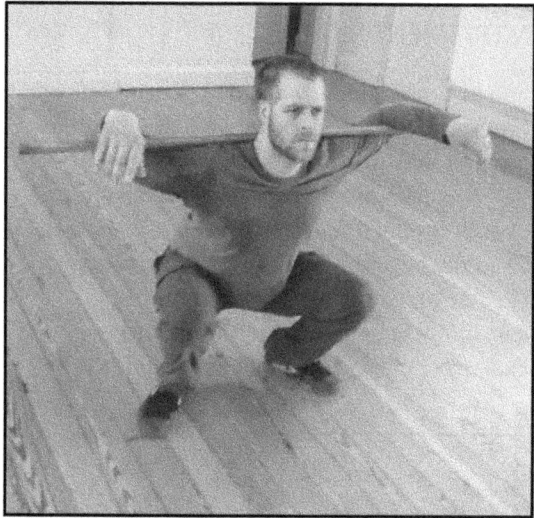
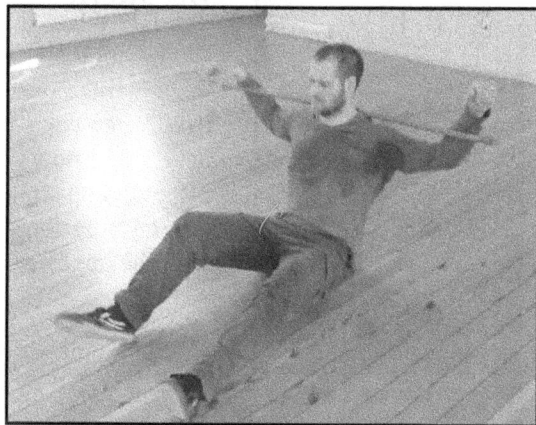
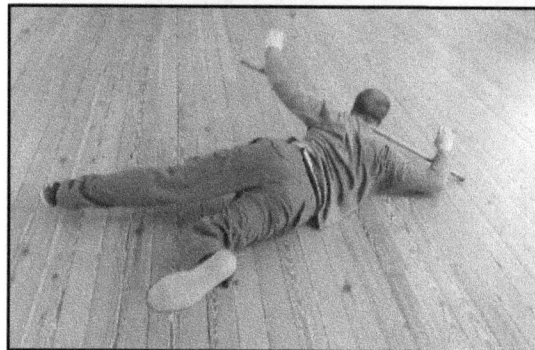

MOVEMENT CHAINS

I've mentioned Movement Chains a few times, so let's take a closer look at what they are and how to create them.

A Movement Chain is basically a series of exercises joined together. There is no pause, you flow between one exercise and the next. Let's begin with a specific method of transitioning between the three Core Exercises. We will combine the squat, the push up and the Mountain Climb in order to make one exercise to work the upper, middle and lower body.

You will sometimes see this exercise called Burpees or the Squat Thrust. A jump can be added in at the end point if you wish. However, as always, our emphasis, especially at first, is on good posture and smooth movement throughout the whole exercise rather than blasting reps.

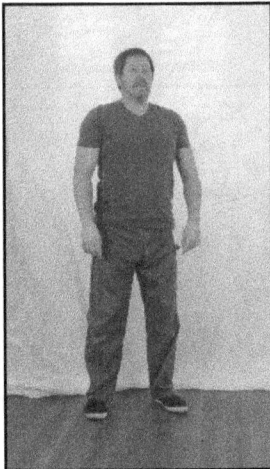

THE SQUAT THRUST CHAIN

I recommend that at first you just run through the movements slowly in order to get the sequence firmly fixed. Then you can begin to pick up speed until you have a nice flow going.

Stand up straight and take a few breaths. When you are ready perform a single squat, down and then up with the appropriate breathing.

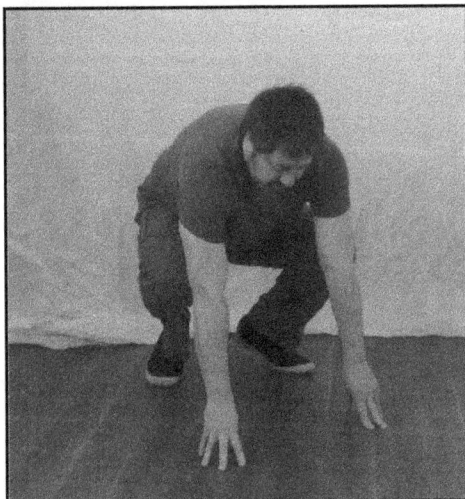

Drop down again, this time into a Cossack squat. Lean forward and bring the fingers to the floor

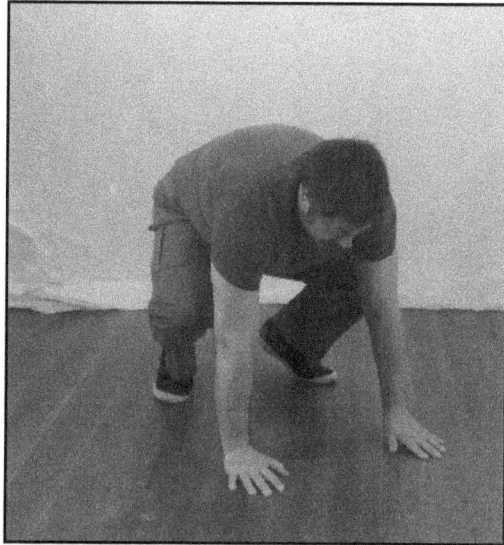

Now place the palms fully on the floor. Lift the hips a little and slide or thrust the feet back. Make sure to keep the shoulders relaxed.

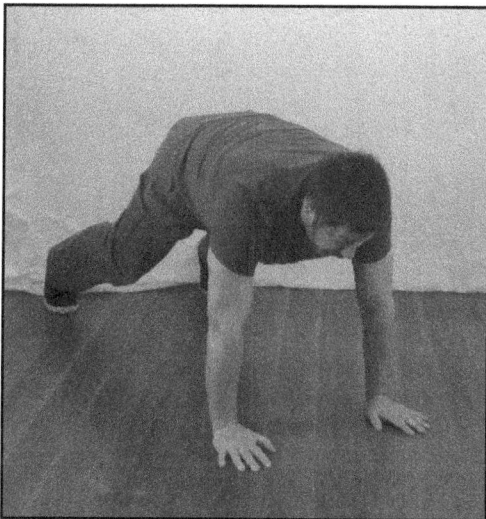

You should now be in push up position. Perform a single push up. We will then go into the Mountain Climb.

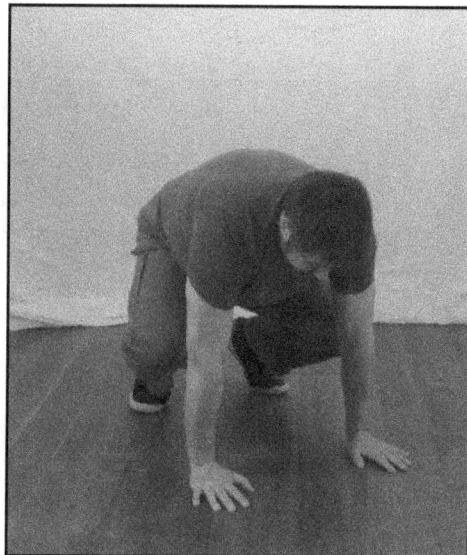

Singly, or both at the same time, bring the knees up to the chest, then thrust back again. To get up, bring knees forward once more, rock back into Cossack squat, then stand up.

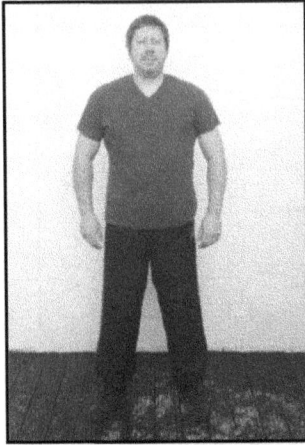

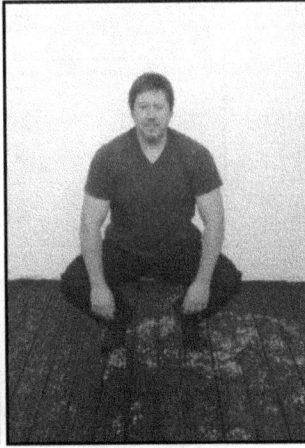

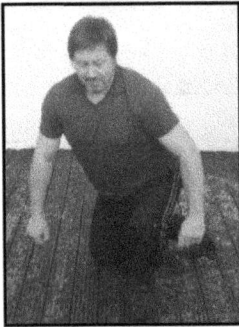

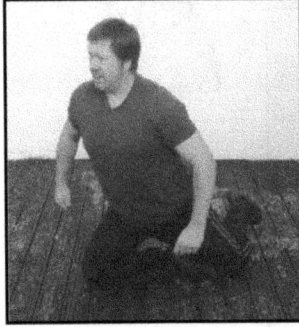

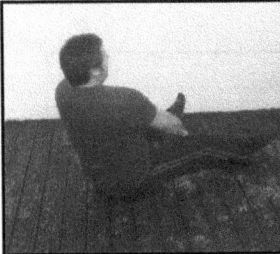

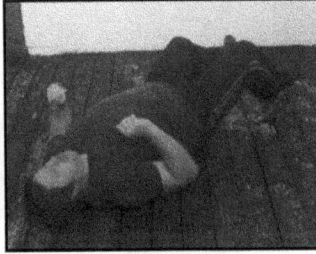

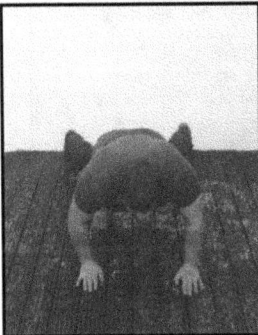

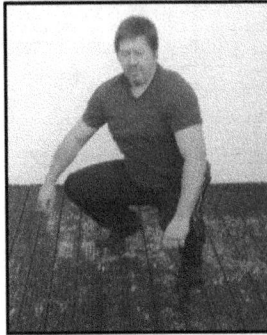

So that's the basic procedure. You can try it two ways. You can rotate through each movement a single time, counting the whole routine as one movement. Or, you can perform a set amount of each part. So five squats, five push ups, fives MC's , five jumps and so on.

You can try the same thing with pretty much any sequence of exercises. This is particularly true of the ground movement exercises, where a side roll flows easily into a back roll and so on. You can start with something quite simple, here is an example.

From standing, go into Cossack squat. Transition into Knee Walks. When ready, sit and do three back rolls. Now do three forward rolls, ending up face down.

Get into push up position and perform push up rolls to each side to get back onto your front again. From there, bring the knees up, work into Cossack squat and stand up to finish.

So that is a group of individual movements combined into one "chain". You can easily put together more and, over time, you can be continuously moving for five or ten minutes.

As always, pay attention to breathing and posture and do not rush the movements. If you find there are points where your movement gets a little stuck, or you have to rush through to complete, then repeat that part and try and pinpoint the problem. It's good for you to develop you own way of transitioning between exercises, be creative in your thinking!

WALKING & RUNNING

Walking and running are easy exercises to fit into our routine. The average person in the UK walks around three to four thousand steps a day. If we can increase that to seven to ten thousand a day, the health and fitness benefits are quite marked. So the first thing to do is examine your daily routine to see if you can include more walking. If practical, can you get off the bus or train a stop earlier and walk the rest? You could try taking the stairs instead of the lift. In your spare time, get out to a nice spot for a scenic walk or ramble. Of course, if you have a dog you may well be doing enough walking anyway!

Running may be a little more difficult as you will usually need appropriate clothing and a shower afterwards. So jogging to work may be only be possible if you can change/shower once there. Jogging, then, is usually something we have to specifically set time aside for. If you can, fitting in even a ten minute jog once a week is a good start. Set yourself a manageable distance, say once round the park, and off you go.

There are entire books written on the bio-mechanics of walking and running. Suffice it to say, be mindful of the Four Pillars and you won't go far wrong. The main issue is how you use the hips in order to minimise impact on the lower back and knees. So be sure to keep your hips relaxed, lift the foot by rotating the hip rather than through

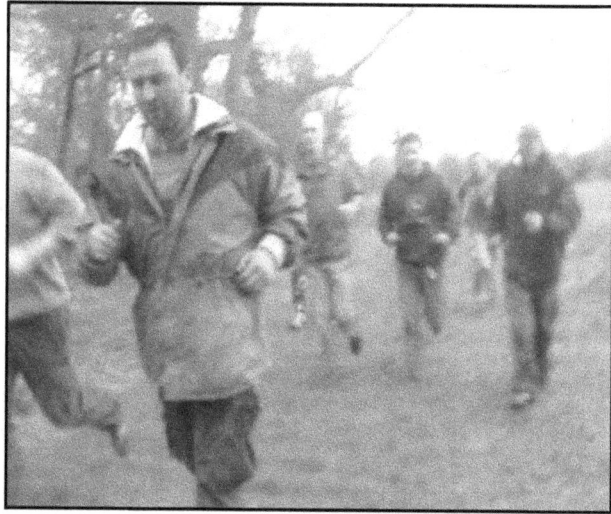

tension. Also be aware of your shoulders, neck and face. I see a lot of people running while hunched up shoulders and grimacing, a sure sign of too much tension and poor breathing. We've already discussed some of the breathing patterns you can add into your walking or running, the most basic idea being to establish a smooth inhale/exhale rhythm that will feed into your overall speed.

Before starting, it's a good idea to warm up. A few leg movements for a walk, or five minutes stretching for a run. It's also good to stretch/warm down at the end of a long run, to rid the muscles of any residual tension.

Clothing should be appropriate to conditions, especially your footwear. Don't shy away from being outside when the weather is poor, there is something refreshing about running in the rain or on a cold,crisp morning. Personally, I'd run in the rain any day over being on an indoor treadmill under fluorescent lights.

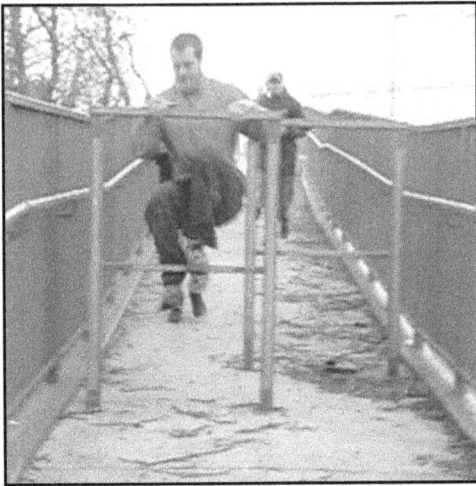

Hydration has become a big issue these days. It's not uncommon to see walkers and joggers clutching water bottles as they move. To be honest, if you are an averagely hydrated person and have no medical issues, a jog without water is not going to do you any harm at all. So don't feel you have to take a gulp every twenty paces - you don't. Drink sensibly at the end of any exercise and you will be fine. I tend to avoid "sports drinks" too, plain old water works just fine, or a peppermint tea if you want some flavour!

We can, of course, apply our Formula to walking and running too. Speed is an obvious variant, but think also of posture. Try walking on different parts of the feet- the heels, the outsides, etc, you will find it engages different muscles in the leg. You may not want to try this in public, though! Try landing the foot heel first and toe first (like a gliding movement.) If you want to test your spinal

alignment, walk with a book on your head.

Obstacles can be used to go around or over, as with our ground movement. You can use furniture or,if outside, trees or other objects. Just be careful when changing direction at speed, be light on your feet and avoid undue strain on the knees. On our outdoor workshops we often get people to move quickly through woods and forest. Not only does it help with footwork, it also relaxes the upper body as people twist to avoid branches. It promotes good awareness too, just be ware of eye safety, wear protection if necessary.

If you don't have obstacles and want to add in footwork changes,then change direction every set number of steps. Try moving backwards or sideways too (checking what's in the way first!). Again, each will work different muscles in the leg, as well as adding a bit of interest into the exercise.

The final variant for walking is height. Try sinking down into a squat for the duck walk. Best at first to do this with some support and

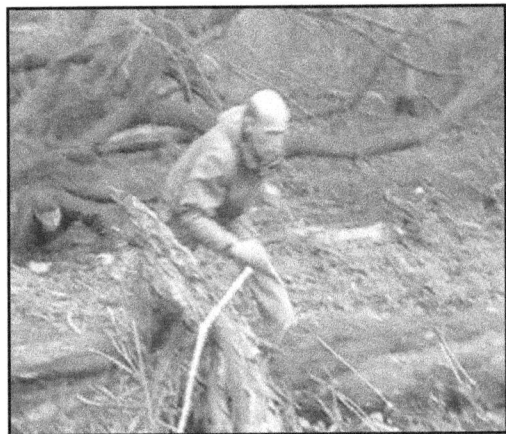

only after you have been working on squats for a while. Try and keep the body upright as, from the squat position, you bring one foot out in front of the other. It is very important here that you rotate from the hips to bring the leg forward. Trying to power from the thigh muscles uses up a lot of energy and you won't get far! Keep a close eye on your knee alignment, breathe and work in increments until you can smoothly take fifty steps in the low squat.

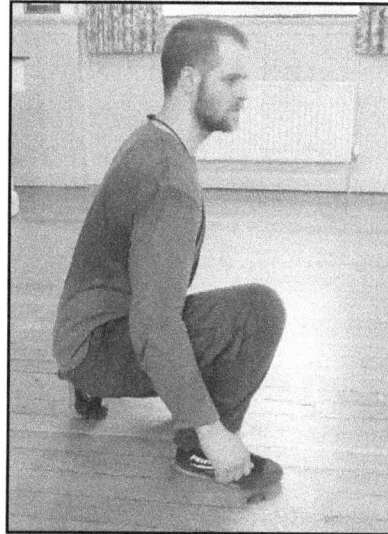

While on the subject of outdoor training, there are, of course, many other activities we can do that will feed back into our fitness and movement training. Climbing, horse-riding, obstacle courses, any activity that involves full body movement and an element of focus and brain power are good for us. You can practice these things in a formal setting, or you can go "off road." Of course, safety is a primary concern, so always be sure to have the right gear and to know what you are doing. Never go solo climbing and always be aware of weather conditions and dress accordingly.

Above all, have fun with your exercise. Even though we have shown only a few basic exercises, the variations and combinations you can get from them should be enough to keep your training sessions fresh and invigorating. Be creative in your approach and once an exercise gets comfortable, always look to adapt it to give yourself a fresh challenge.

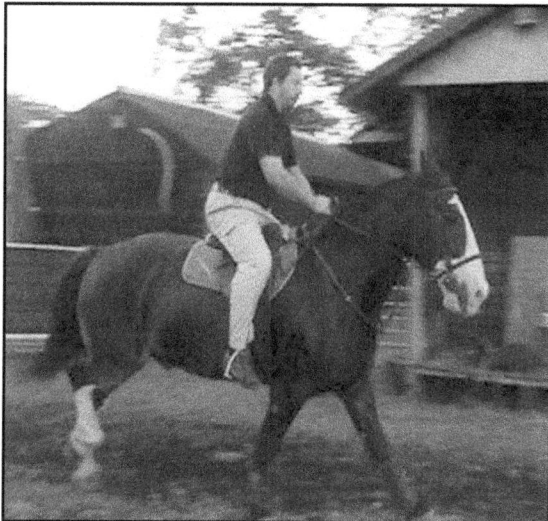

If you have young children, watch how they interact with the world around them. They are constantly exploring, climbing, crawling and using the natural world in order to develop both their physical and mental attributes. There's no reason for that to stop as we get older!

CHAPTER TEN

INTEGRATION

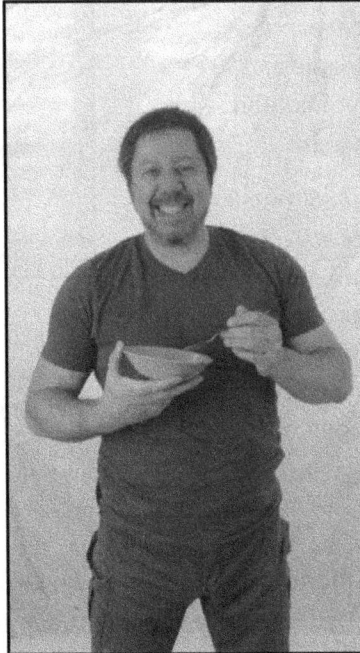

TRAINING

These, then, are our basic exercises and variations. The next question is how to construct a training regime. My personal preference for training is "little and often." Consistency is the key to achieving results, tempered with realistic expectations. So many fitness programs are sold on the basis of chiseling a certain body shape, usually illustrated by a professional model. That model has spent hours in the gym training a daily weight-lifting routine just to develop a specific physique. Those of us with families and busy lives need a different approach - plus we are also working to a different end.

I suggest breaking exercises down into ten minute segments. This way, if you have less time you can just do ten minutes. If you have a little longer, string a few of the ten minute routines together. People in the past new this, and modern sports science is now beginning to catch up, with many new studies finding that those who spent regular time doing a moderate level of exercise expended more energy overall than those who did bursts of high intensity exercise and were then relatively inactive.

Another option is to fill in "dead time" with exercise as and when you get it. Waiting for the kettle to boil?

Ten push ups. Waiting for that huge document to print out at the office? Shoulder rotations. Alongside this, learn to fit the movement exercises into your everyday activities. Don't bend to pick something up that you dropped, squat instead. This way you will develop the idea of exercise as activity.

I find this also helps with motivation. It can be dispiriting to think "I have to go out on a cold night to the gym for a couple of hours."Instead, your work gets done in small packets. Of course, if you have time, there is nothing at all to stop you training longer sessions. I like to go for a thirty minute run at least once a week, then do some stretching when I get back. I'm also teaching regular

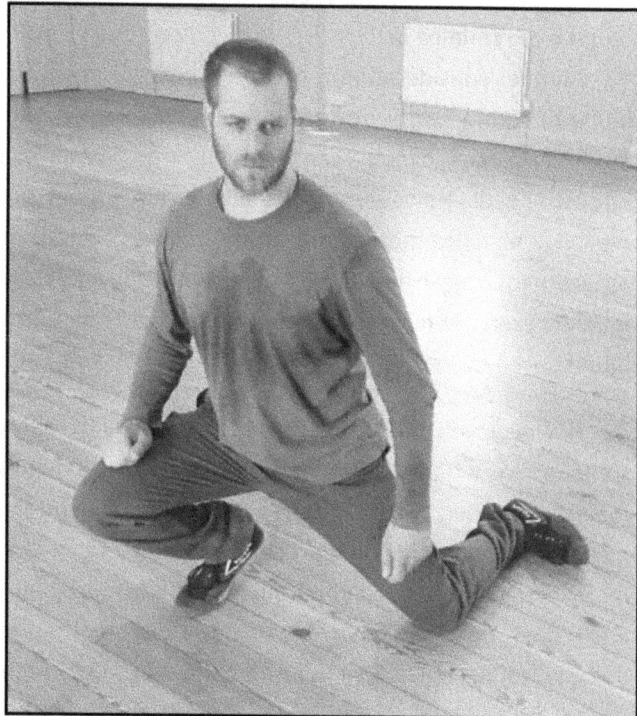

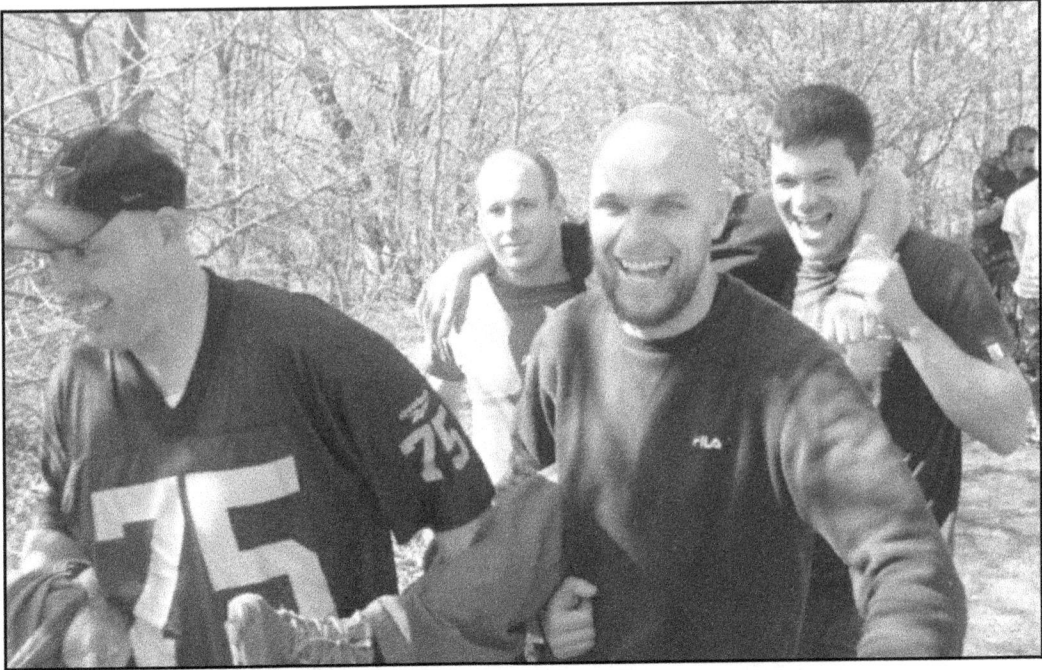

classes each week, which is a good opportunity to get extra training in.

Another consideration is do you practice alone or with a partner or group of friends? Practicing alone means we can focus purely on our own needs. However, practice in a group may give us extra motivation, add a social aspect to training an also give us opportunities for extra exercises (covered in our *Human Gym* book).

However you train, always give yourself some recovery time. Within the session, that means restoring your breathing back to normal before continuing, particularly after a more intense exercise. If you train heavily for a few days, give yourself a day off, or a day doing softer exercise. Give your body time to get rid of any unwanted tension.

At the end of the day, you must find your own balance between time available and commitments, space and opportunity and your own particular aims and goals. Having a goal of achieving X amount of push ups is good, or of being able to bend and tie your shoelaces without groaning! Other times, it's nice to move and train just for the joy of it, with no specific goal in mind.

Of course, there are numerous sports and activities you can take part in too. One of the good things about the *Simply Flow Program* is that the attributes you develop through our training will stand you in good stead in all other activities. Horse riding? Posture, core strength, relaxation. Tennis or golf? Flexibility in shoulders and hips, stamina. Ballroom dancing? Posture, poise and and flow. Even simpler things - a kick around with your grand kids in the park, a long walk, swimming when on holiday - will all be enhanced by our training.

STRESS

There are other, less tangible benefits to training, too. Martial artists have known for generations the importance of a clear and focused mind. As mentioned before, when you train with breathing as guiding principle, your movement become mindful, which will also carry over into your daily activities.

Stress is a major cause of illness and work days lost in the UK. Learning to manage it is perhaps the biggest benefit of all - whether you are waiting to go in for an important interview or just suffering life's stresses in general, these methods will help considerably.

The guiding principle with any kind of tension, physical or psychological, is to deal with the issue there and then, or at least as soon as possible, don't let tension get a foothold. Of course this is not always easy and we may well have some more deep set tensions from previous experiences. Dealing with those is something we will cover in a future book.

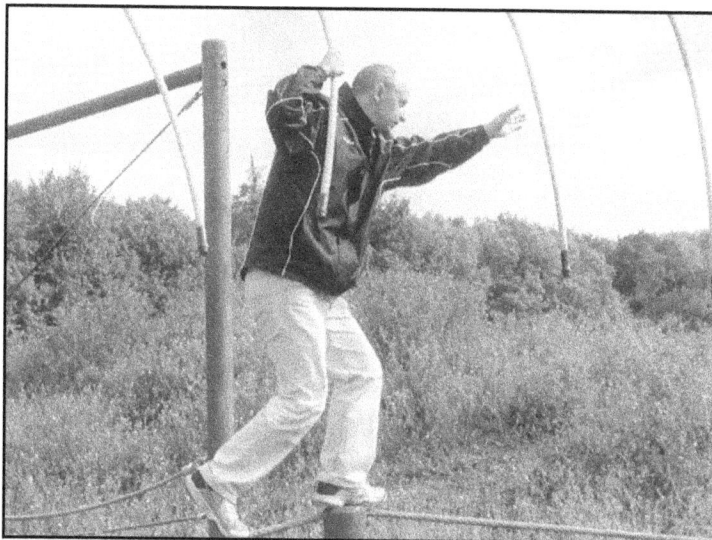

LIFESTYLE

Balance is another important principle. Many martial arts hold that *the key to mastery is balance*. This means balancing not only your training with other aspects of life but balancing all aspects of your life.

The work/family balance can be very tricky at times, especially when under financial pressure. But don't make yourself ill for the sake of earning, nothing is worth your health. Take time out to relax and enjoy yourself. That may be watching a movie, it may be getting a hobby - knitting, making model ships, playing darts - anything that gives you enjoyment for the sake of it.

Arrange regular family activities, date nights with your partner, or activities with

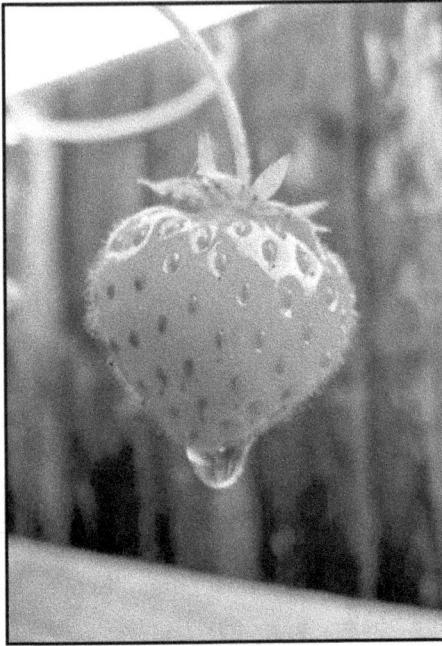

friends. Today s "lifestyle advice" as pushed by the mainstream media centres around having the "right look", buying the latest gadgets, and living the aspirational dream. Learn to manage expectations, don't be too concerned with what other people think, make the most of every situation and live your life to the full, on an emotional level. Be creative and inquisitive rather purely acquisitive. Forge your own path.

DIET

We all know that diet has a huge influence on health and well-being. There are countless diet plans out there, and new trends crop up with increasing regularity. My own personal approach to diet is summed up by

the old saying, "Want to lose weight? Eat less, move around more."

A little simplistic, perhaps, but not a bad place to start. Don't get carried away with this "wonder supplement" or that "wonder diet." Keep your diet simple prepare as many meals from fresh as you can and keep an eye on sugar intake. Do this in tandem with regular exercise and you won't go far wrong.

If you have medical issues such as diabetes, then, of course, follow the guidance of your doctor. But don't feel you have to suffer to get fit! This, to my mind, is one of the most counter-productive aspect of modern diet and exercise fads - the notion that you have to really suffer in order to improve your condition. That approach is all about "the burn" or "smashing goals", diet is about eating two sticks of celery a day and so on. Even if you are doing those things, approach them with a joyous mindset. When exercising, take the air in, feel the blood circulating, enjoy the sensation of moving in the moment. Diet food doesn't have to be plain or boring, plus there is nothing wrong with having a "treat" now and then. Exercise and diet are there to enhance your life, don't become a slave to them!

CONCLUSIONS

If and when you feel ready to increase the intensity of your training, it is easy to do so.. Work more reps, increase the speed, add in the variations for new challenges. This all calls

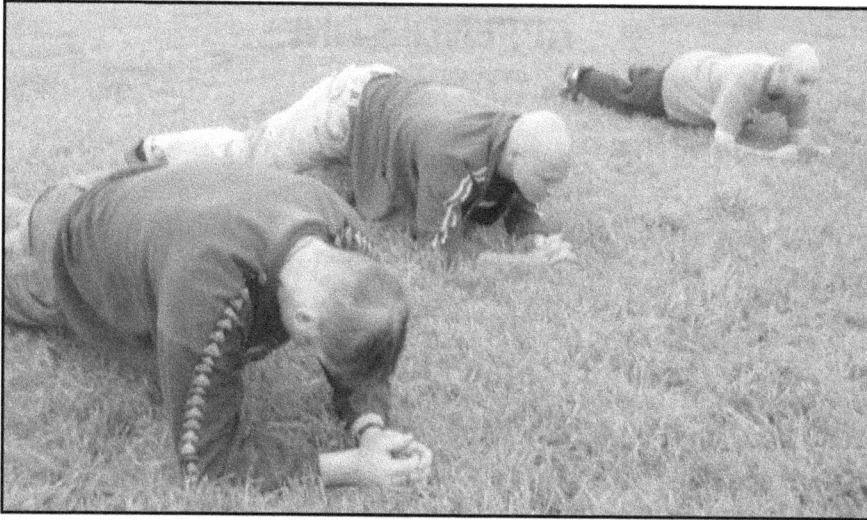

for a measure of self discipline and that varies from person to person. You may be one of those who can push yourself to the required amount each time with no problem. You may be a person who needs a more formalised plan. Sometimes it is good to just do what your body tells you it needs to do. Listen to your body, it is communicating with you all the time! Where is the tension? What feels tight or uncomfortable? Also, at any hint of injury, stop and see a doctor. Similarly, don't be lazy! Three half hearted sit ups once a week will not do achieve anything at all!

To give you some ideas I've put together a number of routines that you can follow. You can also use these as a guide to create your own routines to suit your circumstances. In terms of where to begin, I would suggest starting with some of the breathing exercises, then working through the joint rotation and core exercise movements. From there, you can go on to the stick, the band, the stretching, ground movement and so on. Once comfortable with the basic exercises, start to add in a variation or two. If there is a particular issue that needs more work, then devote some time to it. You may have very tight hips,for example, so put more emphasis on stretching.

I hope this book encourages you to exercise more, but also to exercise effectively and efficiently. If you have any questions please do post on our Facebook group, the details are at the end of the book. Feel free to share your experiences and post any exercise or routine ideas you come up with. Our ethos is very much about sharing and growing together.

The older I get, the more I value mobility. It really is the foundation of all activities. And good mobility means being tension free, balanced and fluid. In short, relax, move breathe, and *Simply Flow…..*

Good luck in your training!

APPENDIX ONE
ROUTINES

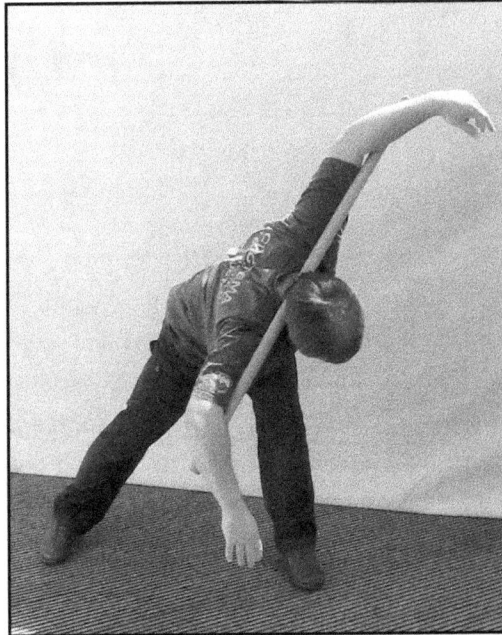

ROUTINES

START THE DAY

Standing, inhale/exhale three times, slow

the breathing a little each time

Inhale and lightly tense the whole body,

exhale relax, three times

Joint rotation - head to legs

10 squats, inhale down, exhale up

10 push ups, inhale down, exhale up

10 sit ups, inhale down, exhale up

Still laying down, inhale tense/exhale relax the whole body, three times

Inhale/exhale with the body relaxed three times

When ready, stand up and start your day!

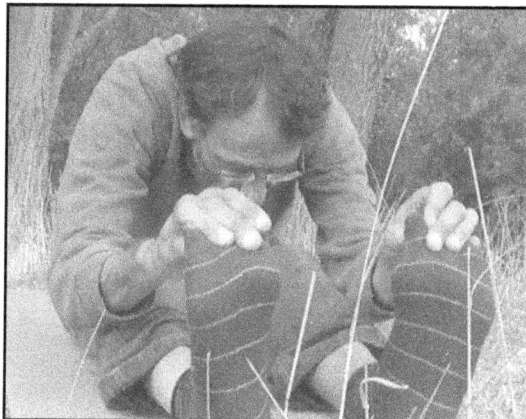

WORKING THE CORE

10 Fall to side

5 backward rolls

10 Mountain Climbers

5 forward rolls

Two minute plank

HIPS

Joint rotation, hips and legs

Ten Cossack squats

One minute Knee Walk

Five minutes leg stretches

ROUTINES

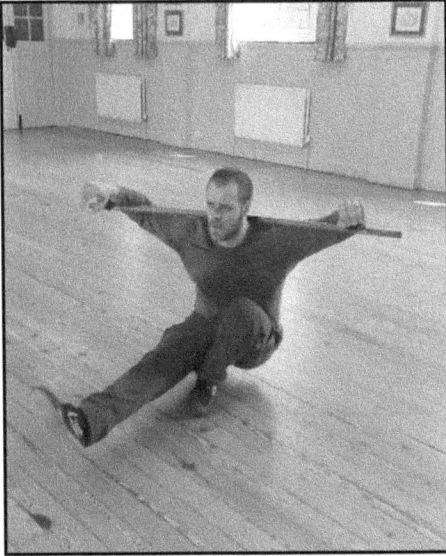

CORE LADDERS

Inhale/exhale three times, relaxed

Repeat with full body tense/relax

Perform one squat, inhale down, exhale up

Drop straight into push up position and perform one push up, inhale down, exhale up

Roll over onto your back and perform one sit up, inhale down, exhale up

Get back up to your feet without using your hands, if possible.

Run through the same procedure, performing two of each movement.

Repeat, this time with three of each.

Now do four. Then three, then two, then one again.

Repeat the initial breathing exercise to finish.

STOP AND GO

10 fast squats

Hold plank position and burst breath until you recover

10 fast push ups

Flip over, hold leg lift and burst breath until you recover

10 fast sit ups

Stand up in half squat and burst breath until you recover

You can repeat the cycle, finish up with static slow breathing

ROUTINES

FULL BODY RELAXATION

Lay down, inhale/exhale a few times, body relaxed. Slow the breathing.

Inhale and tense the legs- just the legs, the rest of the body stays relaxed

Exhale and relax the legs. Repeat three times.

Repeat the same procedure three times with the following parts of the body:

Stomach

Lower back

Chest

Shoulders

Arms

Face and neck

Remember, each time you tense only the selected area, the rest of the body stays relaxed.

Then, inhale and tense the whole body, exhale and relax, three times.

Finally, keep everything totally relaxed and slowly inhale/exhale for a while.

When ready, stretch and move the body around a little before standing up.

LADDER SQUAT

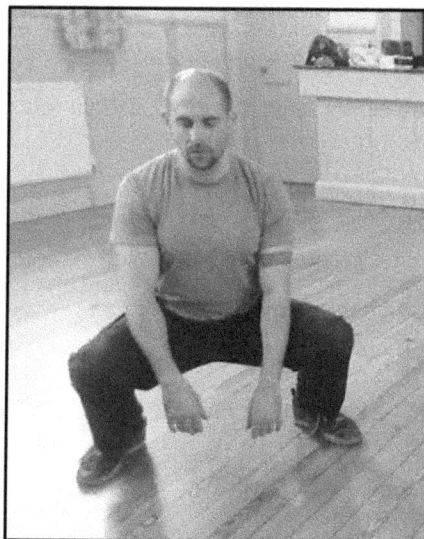

Joint rotation, hips and legs

Perform one squat, inhale down exhale up

One squat on an inhale, one on an exhale

Two squats on an inhale, two on an exhale

Three squats on an inhale, three on an exhale

Four squats on an inhale, four on an exhale

Now go back down the ladder to the single squat

inhale/exhale

ROUTINES

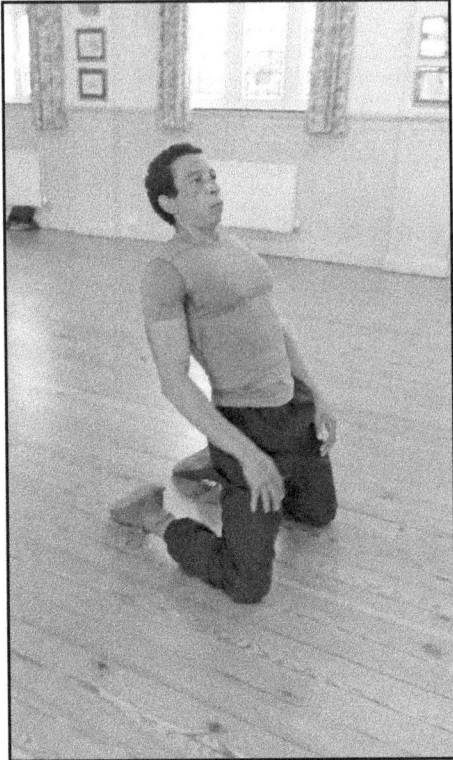

ARM STRENGTH

Standing- inhale/exhale three times, slow the breathing a little each time

Inhale and lightly tense the arms, exhale relax, three times

Joint rotation - neck, shoulders, arms

10 push ups

30 second rest

10 push ups moving hands

30 second rest

10 Dive Bomber push ups

Inhale and lightly tense the arms, exhale relax, three times

Lifting stick above head with tension, front and back

Stick climb un/supported

Joint rotation - neck, shoulders, arms

Inhale and lightly tense the arms, exhale relax, three times

LEG BUILDER

Two minutes static squat against wall

Joint rotation, hips and leg

10 squats

Static Cossack squat one minute

Two minutes knee walking

Two minutes duck walk

ROUTINES

GO SLOW

Squat down to a slow count of 20

At the bottom, put the palms on the floor, move into push-up position

Lower to the floor to a slow count of 20

Roll over onto your back

Sit up to a slow count of 20

Lower down to the same count

Roll over into push up position

Push up to slow count of 20

Draw the feet in to low squat position

Stand to a slow count of 20

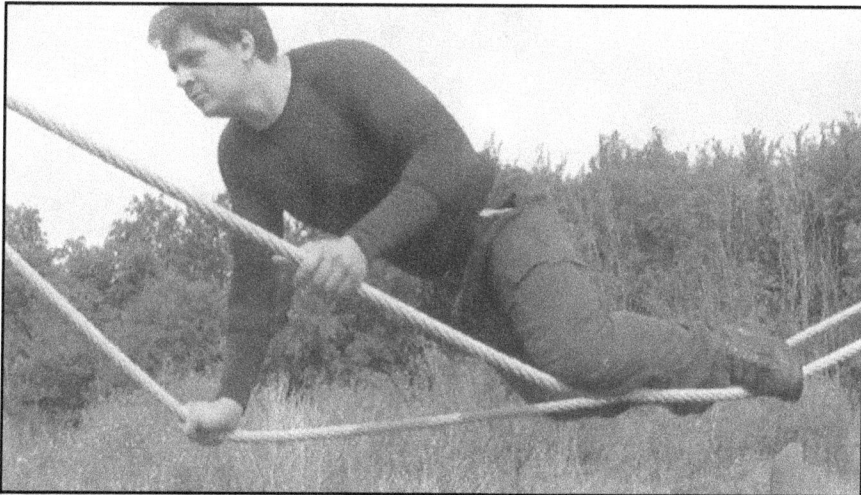

APPENDIX TWO

RESOURCES

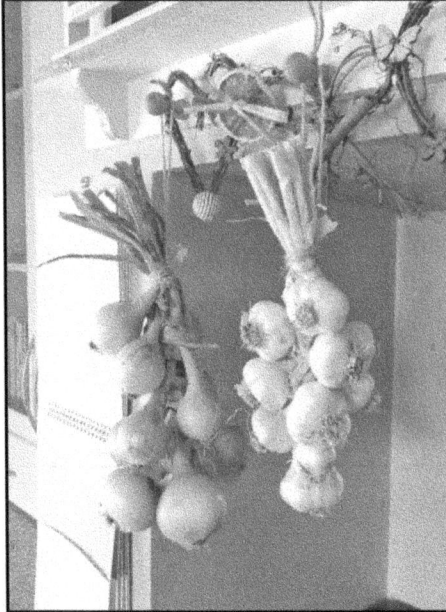

Simply Flow Website	www.simplyflow.co.uk
Simply Flow Facebook	www.facebook.com/simplyflowgroup
E-mail contact	simplyflow@outlook.com
Systema Website	www.systemauk.com
Play Fight	https://play-fight.com
Formless Arts	www.facebook.com/FormlessArts

NOTES

www.ingramcontent.com/pod-product-compliance
Lightning Source LLC
Chambersburg PA
CBHW080625030426
42336CB00018B/3082